AFTER THE DIAGNOSIS

From Crisis to Personal Renewal for
Patients with Chronic Illness

AFTER THE DIAGNOSIS

From Crisis to Personal Renewal for
Patients with Chronic Illness

JoAnn LeMaistre, Ph.D.

Ulysses Press Berkeley, CA

1995

Published by: Ulysses Press
    P.O. Box 3440
    Berkeley, CA 94703-3440

Library of Congress Catalog Card Number: 95-61134

ISBN: 1-56975-046-7

First published as *Beyond Rage* by Alpine Guild

Printed in the USA by the George Banta Company

10 9 8 7 6 5 4 3 2 1

Cover Design: Design Works
Cover Illustration: "Dragon Fly" Diane Ong/Superstock
Editorial and production staff: Doug Lloyd, Jennifer Wilkoff,
    Lee Micheaux, Mark Rosen
Indexer: Sayre Van Young
Color separation: Pro Scan

Distributed in the United States by Publishers Group West and in Canada by Raincoast Books and in Great Brtitain by World Lesiure Marketing

For Jacynth

CONTENTS

INTRODUCTION

My cat was snoring. In recent months, I had had to learn so many new things that I almost could not believe there would be anything left to discover. But here it was. My cat, it seems, snores.

The room was very dark. The cat, very big and black on my pillows. I reached toward the sound of sleep and began to pet her. It seemed I should long since have become accustomed to the change in the way her fur felt to me now. Instead of feeling soft, it felt like pig bristles. I looked toward the ceiling and could not see it. I knew it was daytime and that the lights in the room were on, but I could barely make out the cat's whiskers, so close to my face. I tried wiggling a foot. It seemed to work, so I wiggled both of them. Predictably the cat, now awake, pounced on them. I could not feel a thing.

Once the inventory of physical malfunction began, it seemed to have a life of its own, and I found myself compulsively testing this motor skill and that sensation. Today, I concluded after a while, was not going to be so bad. I could hear, move, and probably taste my next meal. I could not feel anything soft with my hands, however, and the lower half of my body seemed immune to all sensation. The right side of my face had sensations that seemed normal; the left seemed dull. I tried smiling at the cat. I could not tell if she appreciated that I could smile, and I could not see if she smiled back. My eyes were the worst of it, even though I had some sense of light and shape. Eventually, the weird symptoms would clear up and all would return to normal, I comforted myself. I would read, drive, and pet the cat with no changes in my physical functioning.

I hoped some of my friends who had vanished when I became ill would return. I really missed my eyes, but I missed my friends much more, and frankly I did not really understand what had happened. Maybe they thought I was contagious. Many of them were doctors, however, and they would know better than this. Nearly all of them were therapists, and surely they would not deliberately disappoint me or leave me stranded. It was very baffling and extremely depressing.

Almost everything was baffling. After the doctors began taking my early symptoms seriously (and stopped diagnosing my problems as postpartum depression), I learned that I had a baffling illness. The diagnosis was not even assured, because I had not yet had sufficient episodes for certainty, but it seemed likely that I had multiple sclerosis.

I was very fond of my first neurologist—a straight-talking unorthodox man, who later moved away. I had the feeling that the first time he saw me reeling down the hall, supported on both sides, he knew exactly what was going on. There were some lab tests, a spinal tap, and then his summary: Medicine did not have any answers, but he would like me to start on a medication that they thought might lessen the severity of the current difficulty. He was going to treat me as if I had MS. He succinctly explained what he could about the disease, describing the type of scars left on the nerve coverings. He wanted me to see the chief of neurology at a local hospital for consultation, and in the meantime advised rest. What I now had was a nervous system composed of short circuits. "But what causes all this?" I asked. To his credit, he said simply, "No one knows."

The doctor I had consulted at his request was kind and approving of my doctor's reaction to the illness. With a perfectly straight face, he told me medicine was making strides in research and that he wished I had developed the disease ten years later. By then, he thought, there might be better treatment and surely more understanding of the nature of the disease.

Understanding was certainly something I needed to develop. There had to be a way to organize, analyze, and ultimately make sense of the whole mess. I had a six-week-old baby who weighed five pounds. And I was too weak to hold her. I had just finished my training in clinical psychology two weeks before I began dropping things and having trouble with my balance. I was supposed to take the licensing exam, and I could neither read nor hold a pencil. Had I known then—and really understood—that this illness is chronic, I am not quite sure what I would have done. But the doctors had both said every case was different, and that gave me hope. My doctor simply referred to the illness as "the force." Most of the time I felt overmatched and completely at the mercy of this force.

The only thing I could do with ease was use the telephone. This ease came only after I discovered I could actually say to the operator that I was disabled and needed help locating and dialing a number. Before I could bring myself to say I was disabled—and this took nearly a year—I wanted to hurl the phone through the plate-glass window. Mustn't do that— it would wake the baby.

After I mastered the telephone, I discovered a grapevine of people with chronic illness, and I began to call them regularly. I wanted to learn as much as I could from them about how to manage things practically and how to cope emotionally. During my internship, I had had extensive experience with people in chronic pain and had learned a lot from these patients. But now I was the patient, and I found I had a whole lot more to learn. To my surprise, the stories I was hearing all had much in common, regardless of the exact illness. All the people I spoke to had chronic illnesses, and something about the chronicity was important.

By now, I was into the second year of my struggle. By special arrangement, I took and passed the licensing exam with someone who read the test to me and wrote down the answers. I went into therapy to alleviate some of the stress and anger induced by the illness—and by my now ex-husband's reaction to it. I gave a few talks that really lifted my spirits by allowing me to use some of my professional skills. My daughter was healthy and demanding. My strength and stamina were gradually improving, but I was still resting most of the day. Nevertheless, I learned it was possible to do 60 sit-ups a day, and I was walking unaided. By rights, I should have been feeling encouraged, but the depression—caused by anger—was strong and stubborn. I worked harder on my own therapy and began contemplating going back to work.

I was not sure if I could trust my clinical skills. They felt rusty—and I felt emotionally swamped. I began by watching interviews through a two-way mirror, just as I had done as a student. I knew I was back on track when I could predict the advent of a patient's tears from slight changes in the voice. Just as I began to feel encouraged, the unthinkable happened—I got sick again. This time I couldn't walk unaided, and my vision was much worse.

At this point, I began remembering what some of the more experienced patients had told me, namely, that this was likely to be an even more difficult time for me than the first serious bout of illness. The diagnosis of MS was confirmed now, and I was going to have to incorporate that knowledge into my world view. I gave up the fantasy of ever again reading or driving. In fact, I nearly gave up altogether. I was no match for such an insidious, powerful enemy.

The idea of an enemy was something else that in time I had to give up, along with some of the rage the illness caused—at myself and at the world. Being chronically ill is like being assaulted by an unseen and unpredictable malevolent force. But there is a perspective that offers relief from the fear, loss, depression, and anger—the devastating emotional pain of chronic illness. The perspective I want to share with you differs significantly from customary ways of looking at the emotional impact of chronic illness.

Traditionally, the experience of serious illness has been approached in two ways: (1) a gloomy perspective of resignation, self-denial, and helplessness, sometimes unwittingly fostered by our cultural beliefs, or (2) a Pollyanna approach that denies altogether that there has been any real trauma. Both of these perspectives distort and disguise the reality of chronic illness.

The first perspective views the chronically ill person as a failure. This is the patient who does not respond to the "miracle" of modern medicine, and somehow the lack of recovery is often perceived as the patient's fault. This attitude of blame accounts for some of the worst psychological abuse of patients by their health practitioners and caretakers—an attitude typified by the too frequently heard statement, "Stop complaining. You simply must adjust." Unfortunately, sick people may also adopt this punishing attitude toward themselves. Sadly, the word "adjust" too often means "resign," "settle for less than a desirable existence," and "surrender." At its worst, "adjust" is just another way of saying, "You are now a nonperson without the right to experience strong passions, desires, or fierce and unyielding hope." All the anger and blame inherent in this attitude is misdirected: the patient, rather than the disease, becomes the target.

The Pollyanna approach is typified by—and fueled by—personal stories or testimonials of complete recovery from extreme illness or disabling conditions. These stories tug at the heartstrings and catch the fancy of all who read them. Besides creating false hope by overplaying the likelihood of complete recovery, these stories consistently underplay the sadness and feelings of worthlessness that are part of the legacy of any physical or emotional trauma. I do not mean to underestimate the strength and courage of the individuals about whom these stories are written. I intend only to suggest that more than half the story remains untold.

Sometimes, however, it is useful in social situations to present yourself as a Pollyanna. When meeting new people and situations, it may be an advantage for you to let others think you have mastered your disease. The anxiety of other people is reduced by not having to confront illness. The danger is that this Pollyanna image may create a barrier between you and the people who can offer real help. There is no more effective way to isolate yourself than to continually appear self-sufficient, denying any need for help or comfort from others. In short, the resignation viewpoint holds little hope; the Pollyanna viewpoint holds little reality.

The approach I propose took shape as my own understanding developed. My experience as an observer and as a psychotherapist has allowed me to see the many ways in which people creatively adapt and use their individual internal powers of *wholeness* (the sense of being emotionally intact) to reduce the destructive effects of severe physical limitations and the accompanying depression, rage, and fear. The "wellness" approach I present here stresses both the subjective experiences of loss as well as the responsibility for looking outward to reestablish quality in your life.

Central to wellness is the concept of adaptation—the flexible, creative use of resources to maximize your choices and experiences of mastery. This is the key to creating and sustaining a sense of inner tranquility in the face of difficult realities. There is no need to deny the grim facts of existence, or to pretend to others that all is well when inside there is little except torment. To be psychologically well, while physically sick, involves the belief that your personal worth transcends physical limitations; you need positive self-esteem for true adaptation. This belief in your self-worth rarely emerges until what you have lost and grieved for stands second in importance to precious moments of inner peace and joy.

Each stage in the progress toward wellness involves loss, grief, and acknowledgment of internal pain. During difficult times, emotional pain can engulf your life. All sense of time and proportion fade. The scope and intensity of the psychological pain fluctuates day to day. At times, it carries you closer to invaluable inner resources. At times, like a dangerous undertow, this pain drags you far from your recognizable self. There may be a feeling that "I," the person of pre-illness days, no longer exists. It may seem that you have no reason for living or that you are living only to experience pain. Even so, the reason for living is life. The incentive for becoming psychologically well is the potential for the future.

Illness is clearly an emotionally, as well as physically, depriving experience. It can do lasting harm by threatening a person's sense of well-being, competence, and feelings of productivity. At their worst, emotional reactions to illness may culminate in the feeling that life is meaningless. I do not share this belief; but I recognize how stress can make you feel this way.

Illness is a process, and like all processes it has different stages with different characteristics. Sometimes the stages occur in varying orders; often they are repeated. If a sick person lacks emotional support or a necessary feistiness, the process can stagnate, and one may be mired in some phase of the emotional transitions taking place. If this stagnation occurs within a family, some of the less adaptive feelings may cause mutual lack of support and misunderstanding—a tragedy encountered all too often.

You must also realize that the emotional process begun by illness is a highly varied and individual one. Not everyone gets bogged down, and not everyone experiences all the stages I shall mention. These stages are not part of a once-through program, but are repeated as symptoms recur or other losses come about. The level of adaptation is an upward spiral in which coping mechanisms learned at one time can be combined with strategies learned during another time, making each bout of illness less emotionally upheaving.

How people react to chronic illness depends on many conditions, three of which are especially noteworthy. The first is the severity of the illness. The very sick must put their energy into healing, and may not have the luxury of energy left over for emotional growth. The second is the social support available. If you are willing to ask for help and you have a wide support network, you'll have an easier time than if you're isolated. This is, of course, true even when there is no illness in the picture.

The third condition is the pre-illness personality of the sick person. If you've always been pretty resilient, you're likely to have resilience in coping with the trauma induced by illness. The parent who has developed ways of managing the crises of children, for example, or the advertising executive who has learned to deal with unexpected catastrophes in ways that are effective, and not personally depleting, will be able to transfer some of these skills to the unexpected hazards of illness. The salesperson who has counted on a sense of humor to ease job stress will most of the time continue to benefit from it; this asset need not be changed by illness and will aid recovery.

The emotional trauma of chronic physical illness is caused by the loss of a valued level of functioning: a concrete ability such as driving, or a belief that you were on the way to a successful career as a dancer. The chronically ill person not only suffers the loss of immediate competency, but is deprived of an expectable future. No one's future is ever guaranteed, but most people become accustomed to looking at the odds. If I were to attend cosmetology school, for example, I would realize that my knowledge and skills would not help me become a doctor, but I could reasonably expect to be able to find a job in my field after graduation. The formula is, then, if I invest my energies in a particular direction, I can be reasonably certain I'll reach a desired goal in that direction. When illness intervenes, the formula is changed dramatically. All past efforts may seem irrelevant—and in fact they may be. If I had been an artist, the loss of my eyesight would have meant something quite different to me than it actually has.

In the face of such losses, to experience fear, anger, depression, and anxiety is normal. It would be abnormal to deny that your health and your life had changed for the worse. Serious emotional difficulties are more often the lot of people who do not acknowledge the emotional stress they feel, and thereby bottle up depression or anxiety until these feelings are so powerful they break through their defenses. By the time an emotion has become this powerful, it is much more difficult to survive its impact without severe scarring.

Is there anything that can help overcome the displacement and depression caused by physical loss and the loss of goals and dreams? I think the answer is an unqualified yes. Aids in this direction include any goal-oriented striving, any experience of mastery, any outside acknowledgment of competence, a well-oiled sense of humor, any experience of joy, and the constant striving toward an inner state of tranquility.

The stages of the ongoing emotional process—in which these aids are of critical importance—I identify as *crisis, isolation, anger, reconstruction, intermittent depression*, and *renewal*. These stages may appear in varying sequences, depending on the course of the illness, but my observations suggest that they are good summary categories for the whirl of emotions triggered by illness.

CRISIS

In illness characterized by a sudden and acute onset of symptoms, it becomes very clear how sick people and their families react differently to the same event. The patient is seriously ill and very frightened. Both psychologically and physically he or she has a decreased ability to respond to others. The sick person's energies are directed inward toward healing, and controlling panic. The support network, on the other hand, is feeling a highly stressful increase in anxiety. The family carries the full responsibility for seeing that medical care is arranged, finances covered, and that children's lives go on with a minimum of disruption.

Part of the family's anxiety is energizing. It spurs them to seek out doctors, information, sources of support. The family feels increased ability to be supportive of the sick member. Indeed, they may feel a need, sometimes an obligation, to be highly supportive of the patient.

Friends sometimes respond by showering the sick person with cards, flowers, and get-well-soon wishes. Unfortunately, much of this attention is misdirected. The very ill person is less able to appreciate these signs of affection than the family would be. If possible, friends should try to respond to the family emergency, being supportive to as many family members as they can. If you've only been a friend of the patient until now, a thoughtful note to the spouse may be an uncustomary gesture, but it will be greatly appreciated. A very sick person may feel brightened by a bouquet of flowers, but the hospital may not allow them in the room. And patients sometimes report feeling burdened by all the thank-you notes that they are unable to send.

Families are burdened with answering phone calls and responding to other inquiries about the patient. They get tired and burned out when it becomes clear that "get well soon" has no relevance to chronic illness. There is an unfortunate imbalance in terms of attention and support from the outset. I would like to see more direct support given to families at these times, in addition to the solicitous care being offered the patient.

During the crisis stage, almost all of the patient's energy and attention are focused on responding to the physical onslaught of the illness. Surviving is the primary concern.

In addition, the patient and family must cope with the fear of an unknown, and unknowable, future. It is all too clear that the comfortable patterns of the past have been shattered. It is not clear at all what may lie ahead.

ISOLATION

In time, the acute nature of the sick person's illness may abate. But total recovery does not occur, and the illness persists. There is a dawning awareness on everyone's part that the situation has become a chronic one. The person experiences fear about his diagnosis if a definite one has been made. There is so much uncertainty about the future that the patient may not be able to sleep at night, and may seem restless and distracted during the day. The lack of an expectable future constitutes a major assault on one's self-image. The family has exhausted itself during the acute phase, and all emotional resources may be depleted. Family members may be aware that they are angry, fearful, and disgusted about the sick member's situation. Both patient and family members retreat into themselves and their thoughts, now haunted by the knowledge that life may never be the same.

Friends also tend to give out at this point—the idea of chronic illness is really terrifying to most people. After an initial burst of energy, whereby friends communicate their caring about the patient, some friends may find it too overwhelming a personal struggle to continue having contact with either the patient or the family. Some people show an astonishing personal strength as they continue helping the sick person and his family—but some patients have been devastated by an apparent lack of concern shown by people for whom they care. I say apparent because often failure to contact the patient does not mean there is no concern. Friends may care but simply don't know how to act.

Clearly, the chronically ill patient needs a friend who is reliable, strong, and emotionally flexible—a friend who can offer them the important nugget of human contact. Not all people can do all things. Fortunately, the chronically ill get a lot of help from their friends in figuring out whom they can count on. Those who are only a phone call away and who make themselves available when asked are worth their weight in gold.

This brings up a much thornier question. How comfortable are you in asking for help? What does it mean to you to have to ask for help? These questions begin to surface during the isolation stage, but actually they are part of everyday living for most chronically ill people. To really feel comfortable allowing others to help you is an art that must be learned and practiced. It is difficult to fully understand that relying on other people when it is necessary does not indicate weakness or failure, but rather an available way in which to control your existence. One of the emotional barriers to asking for help is a strong feeling of guilt about having a disease that makes one need help. During the isolation stage, patients experience many negative feelings about themselves. But the worst is yet to come.

ANGER

The sick person has been suffering severe upset, terror, anxiety, and helplessness. Add to this the sense of injustice, unfairness, and senselessness of being struck down by disease, and the result may be a rage reaction of tremendous proportions. Often the target of this rage is the patient himself. The ultimate, most dangerous, expression of this rage at the self is suicide. Unfortunately, not much is said anywhere about the commonly experienced feelings of despair that may result in the contemplation of suicide.

There are two reasons why the patient selects himself as the target for these feelings of anger and despair. First, it is almost impossible to be furious with fate; there is no external opponent. In order to provide some structure or meaning for what has happened, many people irrationally conclude that they have brought the disease upon themselves by being faulty or wicked in some way. It is difficult to keep clear that it is the disease that introduced the disruption into one's life.

Another reason for suicidal thoughts is that illness breeds a sense of helplessness. A chronic disease cannot be wished away. The disabilities are there to struggle with as part of daily life, and the threat of a major recurrence or increase in symptoms may be a constant anxiety tucked away not far from consciousness. With the feelings that their underlying problems cannot be solved, along with the belief that they themselves are the culprits, many patients suffer intense unhappiness.

Sadly, the patient's feeling of self-blame is greatly reinforced by society. Often families are unable to help because they themselves are angry at the patient. The changes in their lifestyles that have had to be made are directly attributed to the patient and not to the patient's condition. In families where problems predated the illness, old issues may be raised again with new intensity. Even supposedly neutral medical personnel may be furious with the patient for having a chronic condition. The whole world is angry. And the anger is usually directed at the ill person. It is a psychologically understandable emotional circumstance, but it is very destructive.

The flirtation with suicide, the patient's worst hazard during the anger stage, is a statement of the extent of one's rage with oneself and with those one cares about. But this flirtation may also represent a way to regain control when one's body, one's feelings, and the emotions of one's family seem out of control. It is an illusory control, and, obviously, a most unsatisfactory control effort. With suicide there is never only one victim; there is also the legacy of pain and trauma for the patient's loved ones. The only effective control is the striving toward emotional health.

Another serious problem of the anger stage is the strain on the family. Families who fare better during this time seem to have certain characteristics in common. One is an understanding that the sick person is not the same entity as the disease. Another is the feeling that the whole family is in a major predicament together and is committed to coming out of it as well as it can.

This does not mean that family members are overly involved with the sick member and the subject of illness. Morbid over-involvement with illness and its difficulties produces a family that recites a daily litany of illness-related woes and does not focus on positive family relationships. The family that copes well strives for balance. Enjoyment of events and of one another offsets the concern about the illness. If it had been family custom to attend the movies once a month, this is resumed as soon as possible, or another family activity substituted, even if it is a while before the sick person can participate. Family members must devise ways to nurture and adequately support each other in order to cope with both the anxiety and the practical life changes accompanying chronic health problems.

Anger is the stage most hazardous to emotional well-being. It is also where the most people get trapped. In cases where there is a slow process of continual adaptation to new life circumstances, anger gives way to reconstruction.

RECONSTRUCTION

The sick person may now be feeling much stronger physically or may have had enough time to begin mastering new living skills. Important decisions or new social contacts may be in the picture. What is common to all of these circumstances is a growing sense of safety based on new competencies. Moods are happier, and the difficulties seem a bit further away. In short, the sick person is learning the possibilities and limits of his new competencies. Friends are selected on the basis of how well they react to the fact of illness. The family establishes new routines—or it dissolves as an emotionally independent unit.

What exactly has been reconstructed? Certainly it's not life as it was before. Instead, it is reconstruction of the sense of oneself as a cohesive, intact entity. The reconstruction takes on many concrete aspects, such as the development of new skills, but their most important value is emotional. When a customary pattern of living has been shattered by illness, the patient fears he is no longer recognizable as a whole being. It is the reemergence of a positive self-image that constitutes reconstruction and is the task of this stage.

INTERMITTENT DEPRESSION

Now that things are looking brighter, everyone is tempted to relax, and may therefore be caught off guard when a significant depression recurs. The elation associated with new skills can give way to new feelings of despair as the patient recalls how much simpler it was to do routine things the old way. Nostalgia and grief may combine to produce sadness and discouragement.

Many people know exactly when they expect to hit these rough spots. Medical appointments and reactions to anniversary dates are notable examples. Seeing a doctor, who confirms your intuition that your condition is worse, often leads to depression. So may the third anniversary of having to give up the car, the first anniversary of a divorce, the tenth anniversary of a parent's death, the time of year the physical problems first occurred—the list is endless. The anniversary of an old grief will rekindle the feelings of loss associated with illness. It may be best to seek counseling during these difficult times as a way of shortening their duration and providing a new understanding of what all the feelings of loss are attached to. New understanding brings new resilience; it does not make the losses go away.

Intermittent depressions consist of two elements. One is the awareness of loss of function that occurs several times a day in the course of ordinary living. But clearly, an amputee does not become depressed each time he is reminded he cannot walk normally. There is a second component involved. If the awareness of loss arouses a distinct image of what life would be like if the amputation had not occurred, and if this fantasy has strong emotional meaning for the person, depression is very likely to ensue. This image of how you would be without the illness I call the *phantom psyche*.

The phantom psyche is usually not far from consciousness. It is the self-punishing mechanism whereby the chronically ill person continually erodes his sense of competence or self-worth. "If only I didn't have arthritis, I could still be mountain climbing." "If only" statements are the bread and butter of the phantom psyche. They contain harsh judgments of worthlessness. In a happier mood, you might experience the same feeling of loss, but say to yourself, "I really miss mountain climbing, but at least I can take a walk today."

When the phantom stalks, the soul is very uneasy. Doctors and friends often mistake for self-pity the desperate pain of knowing one's hopeful fantasies will not be realized. "Just stop feeling sorry for yourself" so completely misses the point that it is tragic. It's very difficult to have much sense of self when you're depressed and are afraid that you'll never again be of value to yourself or others.

Self-esteem increases proportionally to successful experiences of independence and purpose, whether the success is remembering what time to take certain medications or walking better after months of physical therapy. The phantom psyche—those unrealistic expectations for yourself—cannot compete with the heady gratification of hard-won success. If family, friends, and medical personnel can appreciate the triumph in being able to struggle, you feel even more triumphant. Well-wishers too often make the mistake of praising a sick person for progress without acknowledging how difficult the ongoing battle is against the inertia of progressive disease.

RENEWAL

In fact, the losses and sadness they cause never go away entirely. Rather, there is a sense of lingering regret for all the capacities that have been lost. A woman who has mastered the technique of using a wheelchair can feel very proud of this achievement and know full well that the device is essential for retaining an active life. But she does not have to like it. When people say, "Just be glad you can still get around," they might be surprised to learn that this comment is offensive. Of course, it is desirable to still get around, but the simple fact is most people in wheelchairs would rather be walking.

It is not necessary to like or resign yourself to the compromises you need to make to get on with living. It is only necessary to acknowledge that changes in lifestyle and skills have to be made. Acknowledging that your skills are different from your pre-illness days is not the same as "adjusting" to illness. There is no surrender involved, only growth—the creation of continued options through new means.

The truly handicapped of the world are those who suffer from emotional limitations that make it impossible to use the capacities and controls they possess. If you have a chronic disease, you need not be emotionally handicapped if you continually strive to become able-hearted. Able-heartedness is within the grasp of all of us. I don't think of able-heartedness as a permanent, static state, however. Developing and maintaining this quality is a process that ebbs and flows, depending on how helpless you feel. Even if you feel in the grip of hopelessness, you are behaving in an able-hearted way by any expression of interest in another person. Shared interest and compassion is what establishes meaning and purpose in life.

When you feel discouraged, you feel all alone—and there is some truth to this feeling. But in many important ways you are not alone. There are hundreds of people in your city who have similar feelings at times. If disturbing thoughts wake you in the night, know there are others also struggling with their pain. And know that if I am awake, I may be thinking of all of us, and of how to make tomorrow come more quickly. No one can share your unique experience, but there is kinship and a strength among those who find it amazing that a cat can snore.

The people I present in the following chapters are in varying stages of the struggle to maintain emotional wholeness and to enhance the quality of their lives, despite the ravages of serious illness. Their experiences are commentaries on courage, dignity, and human kindness.

CHAPTER ONE

CRISIS

At seven in the morning, it was surprising to find that the waiting room outside the cardiac care unit was nearly full. Paul Adams sipped a steaming cup of coffee and began to mentally rehearse what he needed to do during the day for his daughter and son-in-law. He was glad that he was able to be of help. That was the only good thing he could say about retirement. This morning he had not yet been able to see Karen, and he was feeling very anxious. It seemed he and Bill, his son-in-law, had done nothing but wait for the last three days. The last time he had been in this hospital waiting was to be near his wife while she was dying. Paul was afraid he might begin to cry, so he hurriedly took another sip of coffee.

Only three days ago, life had felt completely under control, and he was enjoying planning a vacation. Then he received a call from Bill. Ordinarily the quiet, precise person one would hope for in an accountant, Bill had lost every shred of composure that morning on the telephone. Paul understood he was to meet Bill at the hospital right away because Karen had had a heart attack.

He saw Bill at the registration desk and walked quickly to him. He could see that Bill was badly shaken; his hands trembled as he filled out various papers. Paul had put his arm around the young man's shoulders, and the two of them withdrew to an uncomfortable vinyl sofa. The clerk who was helping Bill disappeared to check on something after telling the two men not to go too far away. She would call them in a few minutes. And so the waiting began.

Bill told Paul that Karen had felt unwell that morning so he stayed at home a bit later than usual. Karen tried to send him on his way with a show of bravado.

"She began to wash the breakfast dishes, while I went into the hallway to put on my coat. Suddenly, I heard a thump and Karen calling for me. I went back to the kitchen and found her doubled over in pain and trying very hard to catch her breath. She was trying to tell me something, and after the third try, I heard her say 'ambulance.' I called the emergency number for our area and went back to Karen. She was crying and telling me that there was a sharp pain running from her breastbone to a point beneath her shoulder blades. She was almost incoherent. The ambulance came very fast. It seemed that I could not get out of the attendants' way. They moved so quickly I could not tell what was going to happen next. Then one of them was asking me if I wanted to follow them in the car. I couldn't imagine leaving Karen, so I asked to ride with them."

Bill was trembling violently as he relived his fear.

"Have the doctors said anything?" Paul asked.

"No. All they said was that they would be with Karen quite a while and I should check her in and then go back to the emergency room. I called you as soon as I got to the front desk."

"William Merton?" called the clerk.

"Yes," replied Bill.

"Everything is in order. You may leave now."

Bill looked at Paul, saying "Let's go back to the emergency room."

After they had waited half an hour with no news of Karen, Paul approached the desk and asked how things were going.

"We'll tell you when there is something to report," snapped a pretty nurse. Paul sat down.

He and Bill were both twisting their wedding bands. There seemed little to say, but they huddled close, as if the combined bulk of the two men could fend off the events of that morning.

Paul thought about Karen and how full of life she was. She had never given up being a mischievous imp. Her elfishness had always been a comfort to him. He had known from the time she was four that there was a heart murmur that might not be the innocent, harmless kind. Her pediatrician had been very thorough, and Karen had received regular electrocardiograms. Her health history was completely uneventful up until now. Paul Adams wondered if somehow he and his wife had overlooked something that might have prevented today's attack. He really did not think so. They had always listened carefully to the doctors. Paul felt doctors were a bit magical. They seemed to have so many answers. He felt confident they would take care of Karen. Then he was jolted by an ugly, angry thought—the doctors had not saved Karen's mother—and she had died following a massive heart attack at the age of 49.

His wife had died ten years ago. It was not possible he was losing Karen as well! Paul was relieved when Bill interrupted his thoughts to tell him he was going to check at the desk once more. Paul smiled weakly in response and watched Bill walk toward the desk with smart, purposeful steps. Whatever they would learn, he and Bill would be in it together.

"There must be something" Bill was saying in exasperation. "It's been almost three hours since she was admitted. Isn't there anyone I can speak to?"

Mr. Adams could not hear the nurse's reply. When Bill returned, he was flushed with anger.

"I'm going to call our internist and see if he can find out what the situation is."

Bill walked to the public telephone across from the nurses' station. Beneath his anger at the emergency room nurse, he felt real despair. They had his wife in another room where he was not allowed to see her, and no one would tell him if she were dead or alive. His hands were clenched, and the one holding the receiver was beginning to ache. He calmed down a bit when a familiar voice came on the line.

"Dr. Cohen's office."

"Vicky?"

"Yes."

"This is Bill Merton. May I speak to Dr. Cohen? It's urgent. "

"He's with a patient, but—"

Bill did not let her finish the sentence. "I really must speak to him."

"Are you all right?" Vicky's tone was professional but concerned.

"Yes—that is, no. I'm fine, but Karen—Vicky, I'm at the hospital. Karen has had a heart attack, I think, and no one will tell me what is going on."

Vicky cut in quickly, saying, "I'll get Dr. Cohen right away."

Bill's sigh of relief was audible. He tried to organize his thoughts so that he could present what he could to Dr. Cohen in a factual manner. Usually, this kind of clarity and organization was one of Bill's real strong points. But today he felt completely muddled. He was reassured by Dr. Cohen's strong voice.

"Bill? What can I do to help?"

Thank God, Bill thought, someone understood he was screaming for help. He told Dr. Cohen of Karen's collapse and that it had been hours since he had been told how she was.

"Let me call the hospital, Bill. A resident I know well may be on duty. He can find out what is going on. Give me your phone number and I'll call you back."

Almost immediately after Bill hung up, he heard the phone at the desk begin to ring. The nurse shot a peevish glance in his direction—Bill felt like the enemy. He did not want to be at war with the medical establishment, he just wanted to know how his wife was. Several minutes passed, and Bill was startled when the phone in front of him demanded his attention.

"Hello?"

"It's Dr. Cohen, Bill. The fellow I told you about will be talking to you soon. You should not have been made to wait this long without some support, if not information.

"This resident? Is he a doctor? Can I trust him?"

Dr. Cohen was saying something about how a resident was a doctor receiving advanced specialty training. Bill was not really following.

Even though he still felt confused about the hospital pecking order, Bill felt he could trust Dr. Cohen's friend. He also felt slightly victorious. The nurse had shoved him around, and Dr. Cohen had put her in her place. Bill did not know it was her fourteenth consecutive hour of work and that she had been asked to remain on duty when her replacement suddenly became ill.

Bill told Paul that they would soon have some information. He felt weak and very, very tired. The nurse was still glaring at him intermittently. Suddenly, he was very sorry the only way he could protect his wife was to become so angry. He did not like being angry, and he especially did not like being frightened. At least when he felt angry, he was not actively experiencing panic.

They were approached by a fresh-faced young man in a rumpled white lab coat.

"Mr. Merton?" He smiled and extended his hand as Bill stood up.

"I understand you are very anxious about your wife. Perhaps you'll feel better if we can talk. I'm Dr. Smythe. Dr. Cohen asked me to help you."

Bill introduced himself and his father-in-law.

Addressing both men, Dr. Smythe began.

"Karen has had a very serious heart attack. They have been waiting to move her to her room until she appeared to be stable and feeling a little better. It was tricky, apparently, at the beginning, but her doctors down here are ready to release her to the cardiac care unit upstairs."

"She's going to be all right, then?" Paul asked.

"At the moment, the outlook is promising. She's had a very rough time. She's going to look very ill when you see her in a little while, so try not to let that upset you too much. The truth is that we really do not know yet how things are going to be for Karen, but her age and good general physical health should greatly help her recovery."

Bill felt exultant. Karen was going to be fine. It probably would not take her long to recover, and their lives would go on as before. Bill turned to his father-in-law and with alarm saw that Paul was not smiling. Instead, he seemed to have shrunk—he was much more stooped over than usual.

Dr. Smythe also saw the anguish expressed by Paul's posture, and he felt slightly irritated. He could not have said any more honestly and calmly that they were just going to have to wait and see how things went for Karen. Paul Adams had seemed like a strong, solid man, and he had not expected his words to come as a blow to him. Dr. Smythe stifled the momentary anger. Expressing concern, he asked if Paul were all right. Would he like to ask any questions? Was there anything more Dr. Smythe could do for them?

Paul heard Dr. Smythe's words and realized he must seem quite fragile. He did feel very vulnerable. His wife had had a series of heart attacks spanning almost ten years. A doctor had said nearly the same thing to him following her first episode. Karen was only 27 years old. Her life should just be beginning. And now they would have to wait and see. See what? This kind of thinking was not going to help Karen. He straightened up a little.

"It has just been a shock, doctor. I'll be fine."

"If you don't have any questions, I'll go back inside. Do you know your way to the cardiac care unit?"

Bill shook his head no, but Paul nodded assent.

"I want to see Karen," Bill interjected forcefully. "Can I see her now?"

"You can see her when you get to the second floor. You will have to give them time to get her settled."

"No. There has been time enough. I want to see her now."

If Dr. Smythe had not had the call from Dr. Cohen indicating that Bill was a very levelheaded man, he would have insisted that hospital procedures be followed. Instead, he said, "Why don't you come with me. We can all see her briefly before they take her upstairs."

They walked through the double doors leading into the emergency room proper. It was extremely crowded in the corridor. Equipment everywhere and many doctors and nurses for such a small place. They all looked terrifyingly young. On a gurney cart outside a room was a woman. There seemed to be plastic tubing coming from both of her arms and her legs. She was being pushed away from them by a husky attendant in white.

"Just a second, please," Dr. Smythe ordered.

The attendant stopped. Mr. Adams and Bill hesitated behind Dr. Smythe. That could not be Karen, and they did not want to intrude on someone else's misery. Dr. Smythe motioned them forward. Feeling sick with anxiety and revulsion, Bill moved closer and took his wife's limp hand. Karen's eyes opened a bit wider, and Bill squeezed her hand.

"We are going to meet you upstairs, honey." Bill wanted to say more, but his voice thickened with tears, so he cleared his throat instead. Paul was stroking his daughter's hair which lay in a damp, unkempt pile on her pillow.

"I'm here, cookie pie." Something like a laugh came from Karen, and Paul realized he had not used this endearment since she was a very little girl. He was glad it pleased her, but he was concerned that he could have said something without knowing what he was about to say. "See you soon," Paul said gently.

Dr. Smythe walked them to the exit. The attendant was pushing Karen into an elevator at the other end of the corridor.

Karen had been having the strangest dream. It was almost like real life, but terribly disjointed. She dreamt she and Bill were having breakfast before she went to her job as a sales representative in the town's most fashionable department store. Suddenly there were lights, unfamiliar faces, lots of loud talking, and the incessant yowling of a cat. There was the sensation of swift movement. Then there were the lights again, and someone was tying pieces of yarn to her arms.

She was frightened—she thought, "I am going to die." This thought recurred over and over again. It made her anxious, but in an oddly detached way. Then the scene shifted to her childhood and her father was tucking her in and saying goodnight. What was that crazy nickname he used? Butterscotch? She couldn't remember.

She was having an awfully hard time waking up. Something was going on because she heard voices again, and something bit her arm as she tried to struggle to consciousness. Now she was feeling more afraid than ever. Something was dreadfully wrong. When she drew in her breath, it felt like something heavy was sitting on her chest and forcing the air out of her lungs faster than she could take it in. This weight was stubborn. There were other body sensations that weren't right either. Something was tickling her nostrils. It felt like there was a strong breeze. She felt tied down, her forearms were stiff, and from somewhere deep inside, there was a yawning, screaming pain that was about to swallow her whole.

As she gained full consciousness, she recognized that she was trying to scream with the pain. She took in the intravenous bottles dripping liquid into her arms, saw the catheter line trailing from beneath the bedclothes. She saw white walls and a bed with rails and gradually realized she was in the hospital. She also saw a maid exiting the room with a mop. She heard a series of clicks and beeps coming from somewhere over her head. There were the low tones of voices involved in quiet conversation outside her door. She felt desolate, all alone. Not quite—she brightened when she saw the toe of a man's dark shoe tapping impatiently just beyond her open door.

The conversation stopped, and in walked a strange doctor. He looked tired, but was a distinguished enough gentleman. She tried to smile, but her mouth was so dry, and besides she hurt so much. The pain isn't quite so bad now, she mused. In fact she felt a little drunk and giddy.

"Hello, Karen," said the doctor as he adjusted something on the board holding her right arm. I'm Dr. Goff. No bad jokes about you're getting the gaff."

Karen snorted her amusement. Her sharp intake of breath when she tried to laugh was enough to begin the agony all over again. There were tears running down her face, but the doctor did not seem to notice. Her nose was beginning to run, and she felt totally unable to fend for herself.

"You have had a heart attack. You are in the cardiac care unit of the hospital. Did you know that?"

"No. I'm late for work."

"That you are. You're going to have an unplanned vacation from work for a while." Karen would remember that phrase for as long as she lived. Is that how people thought of a disaster like this? An unplanned vacation?

"I generally don't cry on vacation. Isn't there anything you can do for this pain? It's awful." No sooner had she said that, than she began to retch. How humiliating! She was going to throw up all over herself.

The doctor, pleasant but aloof, placed a paper pan where it would be useful if she threw up. "You must try to take it easy. We've given you a great deal of medication and your stomach may not like it. We won't let you have anything by mouth for a while." Standing up to leave, he indicated he would return and spoke quickly to the nurse, whom Karen had not noticed until now.

"Stay with her for a while, and keep her head elevated. Keep her visitors to a maximum of five minutes an hour. I want her to rest."

"Can she see her family now? Her husband is most anxious to see her."

"Only one member of the family at a time. And only five minutes. I'll tell the husband to come in now while Karen is awake."

Bill came in and looked at the nurse. She did not leave the room, but greeted him kindly enough. He took in the heart monitor, its leads running down to the bed where Karen lay. She looked awful. She seemed to be dozing, but opened her eyes when Bill touched her shoulder.

"Boy, am I glad to see you, Bill. I feel terrible."

"You look like you've had a hard time." Silly thing to say, he thought bitterly, but that was the most tactful remark he could think of. The blue oxygen tubes sitting beneath her nostrils reminded Bill of a horse's bit. When Karen tried to wipe her nose with a shoulder, the nurse leapt to attention and helped her.

"It's so awful not to be able to wipe my nose."

"I'll see to it you do not have to worry about that," Bill replied, glad at last to have something constructive to do.

"I don't feel like I'm going to be all right. What do they say, Bill?"

"They say you are strong and will feel much better in a few days," lied Bill.

"Good." Karen relaxed a little, and Bill stood up to leave.

"Don't go," Karen was clutching one of his fingers tightly.

"You're supposed to have a nap, honey, but Dad and I are just outside. We won't leave you alone." By the time Bill had finished his sentence, Karen no longer seemed to be listening. Bill quietly shut the door behind him on what he hoped was his sleeping, and not unconscious, wife.

Walking back to rejoin Paul, Bill's mind was spinning with plans and calls he must make. Calls—geez, he hadn't even called the office or the store. Where could his mind be?

"I have some calls to make," he told Paul abruptly.

"Wait, Bill. How is Karen? Tell me what she looks like."

"She looks pretty much the same as downstairs, but she is more alert. They have her hooked up to a monitor, and the nurse will be with her for a while. Karen feels lousy and she's scared. They'll let you in in an hour. I've got to make some calls, but can you stay here in case they want to tell us anything?"

"Of course," said the older man. He felt drained of energy, helpless and very sad.

It didn't take long for Bill to return.

"Is there anything that I can help with?" Paul asked. "What calls did you have to make?"

Bill sighed heavily. "I called the office and the store. John can fill in for me this week, but he's scheduled for a trip next week. The store said Karen should not worry; they will send me the papers so that she can go on medical leave. Then I called Dr. Cohen's office to thank them for the help. They want us to keep them posted. I called my folks, and they said they would drive down here if we need them. I called a nurse's registry suggested by Dr. Cohen, too."

"What was that for?"

"Karen does not want to be left alone, and we can't be with her. I promised her there would be someone available to help make her comfortable. Dr. Cohen said one way to do that was to hire a private duty nurse to be in her room. He called the cardiac care unit and they said that would be acceptable, if she was just there for practical nursing duties such as helping with hygiene and grooming. But the actual medical nursing is to be done by the staff nurses. Dr. Cohen explained that was really for Karen's protection, not just routine hospital policy. That way her medical care stays centralized and the lines of responsibility are clear. At any rate, it will make me feel better knowing someone is there to do nothing but be helpful and aware of Karen's needs. It's three nurses a day. I'm glad I followed your advice and took out comprehensive medical insurance when you suggested it. We seemed so young at the time. Who could have guessed this would happen?"

Paul patted Bill's arm. "Why don't you go home, clean up, get something to eat, and bring back something to do or read. We're going to have a lot of time on our hands."

"I'll be home in a few minutes, then. But if you need me, call. Better plan to let the phone ring awhile in case I'm in the shower. I'll stop at that take-out place near here and bring back something edible for both of us. See you no later than two hours from now."

"Fine," replied Paul. "I'll walk part way out with you." On his way back to the lounge, Paul stopped at the gift shop to purchase a book. Then he got a soda from a vending machine and braced himself for a long wait. He located an empty chair near the entrance to the unit, just in case he could snag Dr. Goff and learn anything else.

Paul tried to read, but he could not concentrate. He found he was looking at the waiting room rug. He never could understand why hospitals had to be so ugly. This one was decorated in Early American garish. The rug had swirls of aqua running through a darker blue background. It made him feel seasick. He realized he hated hospitals. He'd always been afraid of them. Even when Karen was born, he'd hated the feeling of physically walking into the hospital. He was glad to see his daughter and visit his wife, of course, and that had been a very happy time. So what was it about hospitals? They gave him the creeps, that was all. They were places where people suffered, and it always made him feel like he would be the next sufferer. How silly. Most people got well. No, he argued with himself. It was not silly. The hospital houses two very different groups. Them and us. They are anyone connected to hospital functioning—doctors, nurses, clerks. We are the ones who suffer, either directly with a physical problem or indirectly when a family member is stricken.

For the first time, he turned his attention to his companions-in-waiting. They were all preoccupied and tense. Paul noticed how carefully they avoided looking directly at one another. A woman Karen's age was crying. She tried to find a tissue in her purse with no luck and left for the washroom. The hospital is so inhuman. There is not even a tissue dispenser for those who wait. Paul began to feel very angry. It was such a small thing, yet no one had thought of it. He planned to bring a box of tissues from home to put on the magazine table. He looked at his watch and realized it was past time to visit Karen. In order to enter the unit, he had to give his name to a clerk who phoned it back to the desk, waited to receive permission, and finally let him in.

Karen was asleep, but fitful. Poor thing, he thought, as he looked at the tangle of tubes and intravenous bottle stands. There was scarcely room to stand by the bedrail. The room was semiprivate. He did not remember Bill saying anything about Karen's roommate, and he later learned the roommate had arrived after Bill departed. The curtain was drawn so she could not be seen, but Paul could hear her moaning and the nurse comforting her. When the woman quieted, so did Karen. Her color seemed somewhat better, but maybe the lights in here were softer than the ones downstairs. She was clearly uncomfortable, but she seemed to be dreaming, and Paul hoped she would pass a quiet night.

Since the nurse was occupied, he could not talk to her. He stayed longer than the allotted few minutes, until the nurse was free, and then asked about his daughter.

"How is she doing?"

"As well as can be expected. She's very uncomfortable. Dr. Goff is due back to look in on her one more time before he leaves for the night. I can tell you more during the next visit. I'm afraid you must leave now."

Paul nodded and told the nurse he appreciated her talking to him.

The cardiac care unit was settling in for the night; he wondered if he would be able to sleep in one of the chairs. He and Bill had dinner, and both of them stayed that night. The nurses were really quite kind. When it became clear that he and Bill meant to visit Karen every hour, whether she was asleep or not, they brought out some blankets to make their stay more comfortable. Dr. Goff had told them before he left that Karen seemed to be stable and that they must try not to worry. They ate breakfast in shifts, and Bill phoned his thanks to Karen's office for the flowers they had sent. When he checked the house later that day, he found more bouquets sitting on the steps. Word had gotten out fast. Karen had always laughed at the gossipy ways of some of her co-workers, but she would enjoy the flowers.

By the end of the second day, both men were exhausted. They needed to develop a strategy for the night vigils. Karen's condition was essentially unchanged, and the nurses were encouraging them to go home to sleep. It was decided that Bill would stay the night, allowing the older man to sleep at home. Paul would rejoin him after breakfast, and Bill would go home to nap. They followed this routine until Karen was well enough to be moved to a different room on yet another floor.

The morning of the third day, after relieving Bill, who just remembered the cat hadn't been fed since Karen's admission, Paul was again studying the offensive rug. He sipped his coffee, made a list of things the practical nurse had asked him to bring for Karen—toothbrush, hairbrush, and other toilet articles—and again surveyed the other occupants of the waiting room. One of the women, a Miss Smith, had brought doughnuts for all, and they were sitting untouched in front of the group of wary strangers. It was a lovely gesture, so even though he was not hungry, he walked over and selected a plain doughnut.

"Aren't you going to have one, Miss Smith?" He knew her name because he had overheard one of the doctors speaking to her about her mother.

"Please call me Barbara."

"I'm Paul Adams." They shook hands, and he sat down near her. "It was nice of you to bring these for everyone."

"It was really a bribe. I can't stand the quiet and I was hoping to engage someone in conversation."

Another woman said, "It's spooky when it's so quiet."

"Exactly," said Barbara.

More people were selecting doughnuts and introducing themselves. The tension in the room was eased until a doctor came out of the unit. He was always grabbed by an anxious relative desiring information. Throughout the day, the people in the waiting room began exchanging stories about their ill relatives. The atmosphere was transformed by the time Bill returned. When he commented on it, Paul explained about Barbara's being willing to extend herself and how that had helped everyone else. Paul was feeling much better. He had really needed the human contact to make the worrying and waiting more bearable. He reflected about how he and Bill had different styles of managing stress. Bill typically got extremely busy with his long lists of things to do. Paul, on the other hand, became temporarily withdrawn and forgetful. The only thing he had remembered to do thus far was to arrange for a loan. Bill did not yet understand how expensive all this was going to be. But Paul had planned to borrow the money just to have it there, in case.

Even though Bill did not think he would need the loan, he had been grateful. That was something that really had not occurred to him. He knew that being middle class, he and Karen were not eligible for any health subsidies. He also had had a number of wealthy clients whose health costs were staggering, but these did not seem to affect their style of living. He thought he had enough put away to avoid any hardship, but maybe he needed some interim accounting of what had been spent so far so that he could plan. Money had never really worried Bill. He was simply interested in its manipulation and growth through investments. Work for him was a marvelous game, and he didn't imagine that making contact with the hospital accounting department would be difficult.

On the fourth day, after settling Karen into her new room and reading her the cards that had come for her, Bill decided to check with the accounting department. He had already figured out that if he took a photocopy of the charges to date and gave it to his insurance agent, he should be able to know rather quickly how much of the hospital bill would be paid by his insurance and how much would represent out-of-pocket expenses to him. He was not prepared for the almost unintelligible bill when he got it. There were flagrant inaccuracies and charges for things he did not know Karen even had, like lotion and her personal thermometer. The thermometer he would pay for, but not for an extra day of charges. Someone had apparently entered the wrong date in the first entry of her chart. It was a struggle of massive proportions to correct this error in the charges. Bill did not know it would take a full two months of correspondence to rectify.

After only four days, Bill was depleted of energy. His very high energy level—most likely produced by anxiety—had given way to fatigue and irritability. His days were disturbed by calls from friends. Everyone wanted to know how Karen was. Only Karen's boss had asked him with any sincerity how he was doing. He thought he would shoot the cat. It kept meowing and asking for food or attention or something. The point was that it wanted something, and Bill had nothing left to give.

"Let me take the cat to my house," Paul offered. "She's good company for me. I know you don't even like cats and have her only because she was Karen's pet when the two of you married. If it's all right, I'll pick her up before I go home tonight."

"Thanks, Dad, that would really help."

Mr. Adams was very thoughtful. When he picked up the cat, he took a look around the house and saw that the refrigerator needed to be cleaned out. After he had cleaned it, he made a grocery list and put it by the refrigerator. He took a copy for himself. He collected the cat, some food, and a few of her toys and packed her into the car. Before he left, he gave the begonias by the door some water and walked next door to Karen's neighbors. He had met them on occasion and knew they had three strapping boys. He rang the bell and a plump woman answered.

"Hello. I'm Paul Adams, Karen's father. We met last summer."

"Of course, Mr. Adams, won't you come in? I understand Karen is ill. How is she?"

Mr. Adams brought her up to date.

"Is there anything we can do?" the neighbor asked. She was an earnest woman, and the question was not idle.

"That's really why I came over. I was wondering if one of your boys could do the yard work while Bill is spending so much time at the hospital. I would be happy to make it a real job with pay."

"That's not necessary," a lanky 13-year-old supplied from over his mother's shoulder. "Karen has always been very nice to me. I'll be happy to do it."

The boy's shy grin was infectious, and the two adults in the doorway smiled along with him.

"That takes care of the yard, but how about food? Is Bill able to cook for himself?"

"I don't think he's eating much," Paul replied.

"That's what I thought. I've frozen individual portions of our dinners the last three nights. May I give them to you?"

"That's really wonderful," said Paul. "I know Bill will be very grateful."

"Tell him not to worry. We always have plenty, and I'll just keep freezing."

Paul went back inside Karen and Bill's house to put the food away. Confident he had done something useful, he drove the angry cat across town.

Karen's nights passed fitfully, and her days were even worse. When she was awake, she felt too groggy and weak to even think clearly, and her simplest physical activity was exhausting. She was especially perturbed by not feeling clean. No sooner would her sponge bath be finished, than the exertion of the smallest movement would set her to sweating again. The practical nurse would bathe her as often as she requested, but she hated to ask. As long as Karen was silent, so was the nurse. The minute Karen asked for anything, the nurse would begin chattering and Karen did not have the energy to listen. She just wanted to be quiet, to drift into the half-conscious realm of total self-absorption. At first when she had done so, she often heard her own thought, "I am going to die" as if it were being spoken by another. It seemed there was another part of her with another voice that would answer, "Maybe not." Karen felt like she was observing a macabre play. She loved the plucky, but very small, part of her that was not ready to give up yet. As she grew stronger the lines of the play changed slightly. She heard, "I feel like I am going to die" and, "You can do better than that" along with other voices: "It hurts" and "I'm so scared." When she was fully awake, she wondered if she were going crazy.

Mustering her courage, she hesitantly told one of her doctors about her fears. She could not remember things, everything seemed to be happening in slow motion, and worst of all were the voices. She felt restless and uneasy. She was so tired, but she could not sleep. The smallest noises were irritating. The doctor had listened carefully and told her that she was describing a medication reaction. She was not going crazy. These symptoms would become milder now that they were lowering the dose of the medication. He warned her that she might at first experience a different set of uncomfortable reactions due to her withdrawal from the drugs.

Karen was glad to have been forewarned when, the following day, she felt like she had been hit by a truck. She could scarcely breathe. As the days passed and her acute discomfort abated somewhat, Karen realized that she had become sensitive to the smallest change in her physical condition and that she worried a great deal each time a new sensation appeared. Was it normal? Did it mean she was having more heart trouble? She became alarmed primarily over insignificant changes, but how could she tell what was important? She asked her father and Bill to help her get explanations from the doctors.

Karen was looking forward to her release. She felt worn out by the incessant noise of the hospital, the glaring lights, and all the people. Since it was a large teaching hospital, her room was regularly filled by doctors leading groups of students on morning rounds. It seemed she had told her life's story to a million people. She was so tired. Why didn't they just leave her alone? She wanted to go home, to be with familiar objects and in charge of making some of her own decisions again. From somewhere deep inside her, she understood that she would need a long time to recover. She even recognized the possibility that she would not feel like her old physical self ever again. Whatever had changed, she felt it with each bit of exertion. It felt almost as if something were broken. She needed to mend, but she worried about how she would be able to do so. Her mother could not heal. Would the same thing happen to her?

That afternoon, a tired family trio conferred with the cardiologist following Karen's progress. He told them that the special X-rays of her heart showed two of her heart valves as very badly damaged. These valves, he went on, could not heal, and their function to a person's well-being was so important that another means had to be used to help Karen feel well again. He recommended surgical repair. Karen was well enough now to have the surgery.

"What if Karen is very careful, rests a lot, doesn't get overly tired, and does all the right things with diet and exercise?" Bill wanted to know.

"Those behaviors will help her recover from surgery, but they will not cure her without the surgery," the doctor replied.

"Tell us about the surgery and what we can expect afterwards," Karen asked. "I can feel that I am not going to be able to get back to normal without some kind of help, but surgery seems kind of overwhelming."

The doctor told them that there was an excellent track record for this surgery when it was performed on basically healthy individuals like Karen. There were risks of course, but these were secondary to the limitation of Karen's life that would be there without the surgery. Karen would not know how much the surgery would help until it had been done. Even if she recovered nearly all of her former level of functioning, Karen would need to follow the recommendations for diet and exercise routinely made for heart patients for the rest of her life.

It boiled down to more waiting and the knowledge that she was no longer just Karen, but was now Karen with heart problems. The doctor had said she was a heart patient. Karen felt that was an attempt to make her less an individual than she had the right to be. As the doctor left to schedule the surgery, there seemed no question that her life had changed radically. She was staggered by the enormity of the job in front of her. She would need to recover from the surgery and rebuild a life for herself. She looked at the two tired men by her bed and wondered if they would be able to help her enough, and if she could do it.

COMMENTARY

Karen's story is typical of situations characterized by an acute onset of symptoms, and where the chronicity of the condition requires major life changes in the future. Her story is, perhaps, unusual only in the extent of the active support of her family. She has a safety net to catch her that may not be present in all cases. Starting with the beginning of the story, there are several general points to highlight.

Each person brings a unique set of experiences, skills, and attitudes to the encounter with physical illness. Each member of this family, as well as the hospital staff, reacted to Karen's heart attack differently, in part because her illness caused each one to have feelings reminiscent of other times in their lives.

Paul Adams, for example, associated the hospital's cardiac care unit with his wife's death, and was stunned by the almost unthinkable awareness that he might also lose his daughter. The threat of loss presented by Karen's attack affected him differently than it did Bill. Paul was more immediately aware of his deep-seated fear than was Bill.

Some people when confronted with their own fears of illness truly panic. For example, in very extreme cases, we read of husbands who desert their families upon learning that their wives are seriously ill. It is easy to judge these actions as despicable, but they really are manifestations of weakness on the part of people overwhelmed by anxiety. Paul Adams did not panic. Rather, he experienced a state of temporary shock that was eased by his characteristic style of coping with anxiety concern for others. He took care of his daughter and Bill, even the cat—everyone but himself. It is often the case that the Paul Adamses of the world with time become depressed.

Paul is usually able to lessen the impact of personal distress by a pattern of friendly problem-solving in the external world. This can be a highly effective way of coping, for it develops strategies to eliminate problems. Borrowing money for Bill and enlisting the help of the neighbor's boy are good examples of such strategies. Paul Adams and others like him are "helpers." They do not ask for help for themselves, and they do not appear angry if other people begin to take them for granted. They seem to desire no acknowledgment—indeed, Paul Adams' thoughtful actions and genuine concern for others will be rewarding in themselves up to a point—but helpers have a strong need to please. The self-esteem of a helper like Paul depends on his unspoken expectation that others will perceive him as being very helpful, that his efforts will gain positive recognition from other people. If, then, other family members should become critical of him, Paul would be likely to feel misunderstood, slighted, and angry. Paul would not express this anger openly, but would use it to castigate himself. This kind of anger when turned against oneself produces marked feelings of sadness and defeat, that is, depression.

The neighbor boy's responsiveness to the request for a gardener is an example of how the social environment can be supportive of people like Paul, who are wrestling with the emotional demands of an acute episode of illness.

Bill's anxiety is more clearly in response to the immediate problem of Karen's health. He felt shattered when he had no clue about what he could do for Karen, but his insistence on being informed about her condition was an appropriate and productive response. He demonstrated resourcefulness in recruiting the aid of the family doctor. This ability to seek and acquire information will be an advantage in the months to come. What will be troublesome to Bill is his strong need for order, predictability, and sameness. This need is suggested by his belief that the doctors will "fix" Karen and that their previous life can be resumed, largely unaffected by this incident of illness. In part, this is simple naiveté; in part, hopeful optimism. But it may also reveal a need to distort reality when the news is grim. Bill's strong need for order helps him manage practical detail, but it may also work against him, for illness is not a tidy, orderly condition. What Karen needs most now may be very difficult and frustrating for Bill, namely, the ability to tolerate the uncertainties and ambiguities that are part of life for the chronically ill and their families.

Bill was in his element when he could make lists of concrete actions to undertake. His relief came from feeling he had accomplished these tasks and that life was going forward. For many people undergoing an emotional crisis, it is extremely useful to be doing something, however small, that they judge to be productive in its own right. Bill's anxiety in the waiting room was beginning to trigger rage at the apparent unresponsiveness of the hospital staff to his need to know how his wife was. If he had been unable to convert this into a productive strategy to get help, it is possible that he would have become overwhelmed with a set of powerful emotions he ordinarily kept under tight control. For Bill, these were anger and anxiety.

The emotional devastation felt by a person flooded with anxiety may lead to his being unable to make any choices at all. If he feels completely trapped in the situation, this loss of perspective can lead to his being unwilling to go home, sleep, or eat for the duration of his relative's hospitalization. For any of these actions require a decision, and being emotionally out of control, he cannot make a decision. Self-esteem erodes daily for these poor people—and you can find them in any hospital. It makes sense to stay close when a relative is newly admitted in fragile condition. But to stay after a condition has stabilized only because one cannot make the decision to go home is self-destructive. At times, one can even detect a bit of unconscious competition with the ill person on the part of a family member who is making himself sick under the guise of taking care of the patient.

Bill and Paul seem to have solved the problem of how to manage the hospital vigil without exhausting themselves, or being overwhelmed with anxiety. Someone was nearly always available to Karen, but they were also able to take care of themselves moderately well.

Unlike Paul, who had a sense for the marathon task ahead, Bill functioned primarily on nervous energy. He did not pay attention to his own nutrition and rest as well as he might have. Amid the many tasks he gave himself, he did not call a friend to confess his fear, or clearly open the door for others to help him. The greatest point of concern for someone like Bill is that there are often no precise steps that can be taken to aid the physical recovery of a loved one. What often is most needed at this stage is the ability to calmly wait with the patient. Often, no words are even needed. The presence of a loved one who is not impatient to leave and who does not convey an unspoken message that the patient's illness is imposing a harsh duty on him, is the greatest comfort of all to a patient who needs help wiping away the tears or blowing her nose. Bill's characteristic style of dealing with life may not allow him to be relaxed with Karen under these conditions, so he did what was comfortable and practical. He arranged for the private nurse. Not everyone has the financial resources to do this, but one can often arrange for a succession of friends to sit quietly with the patient when the hospital permits this.

Karen had to deal with both the terror brought on by a sudden collapse and with her recollection of her mother's illness. But whatever fears she may have experienced as a child because of illness and the loss of her mother, clearly she had also learned that her father was a steady man who would not desert her in a time of need. Her sense of desolation is only transient; she gives no hint that she feels entirely abandoned. Karen's immediate concern is how terrible she feels and whether she will live. A bit later Karen's mood becomes quite introspective. She monitors even very subtle changes in her body and worries about them. Her strength is in her focus on her present condition. She lets Bill handle business, and to some extent, lets the future worry about itself. Her job is here and now. It is her job to recover, and it is a staggering task. For this, she needs information from the doctors about the meaning of her physical sensations and the strange changes in her thoughts. Later, as her fear of death abates, her concern is for the quality of her life; will it be a life she can value?

The reactions of the various staff in the hospital are interesting. For the clerk at the admitting desk, this incident was simply a normal part of her eight-hour-a-day job; the personal concerns of the family members are no concern of hers. If this attitude is couched in respectful behavior, it is completely unobjectionable. If it leads to rude or insensitive behavior, it is highly objectionable and should be reported. The cranky nurse was unprofessional. Her behavior is understandable on the basis of her fatigue, but another equally fatigued nurse might have handled the situation very differently. This nurse's attempt to bully Bill is an inappropriate response, though an all too common one. Bill's reaction of seeking information from a "higher authority" was very effective.

The doctors were all medical professionals first, and human beings second. Our society places a most unfair burden on doctors; they are expected to have the answers, be fresh and alert at all times, and allow us to feel we have been in the presence of a godlike being. No one can live up to these expectations, and no one should have to. On the other hand, the public all too often gives permission to doctors to be arrogant and insensitive. The doctor-patient partnership between skilled doctors, and patients who are willing to provide accurate data is becoming more widespread, but it still has a long way to go. For many years, patients quietly went along with the expectation that they would have no say in the affairs of their bodies. Changing the traditional roles of passive patient and omnipotent doctor into a partnership or shared responsibility will require a period of transition. Doctors and patients need to learn to treat one another with true respect. Doctors must not promise what they cannot deliver, and patients must learn to refrain from asking for it. Both must be able to recognize when they are afraid. Patients who complain of doctors' dealing with them like cars on an assembly line, feel abused by the doctors' apparent lack of connection to them as individuals. When this happens, it is frequently because the doctor is unable to invest much of himself in the patient for fear he will be dragged down by the patient's anxiety—or worse, have to deal with his own fears of mortality.

Patients must perceive that when they become anxious they behave in ways that make them hard to bear. Is the answer, then, that the patient should not be anxious? Of course not, but he should have enough self-knowledge to realize that when anxious, he becomes argumentative or demanding, or inappropriately passive. The ill person who has these self-perceptions, and thus refrains from becoming abusive to the doctor, helps create the conditions for improved medical response to his own needs. Likewise, the doctor should be conscious of his own anxieties and emotional biases. A particularly unproductive bias is the doctor's need for patients to be compliant and pleasant—and to go into remission. Obviously, these are the most gratifying occurrences in a physician's work life, but the doctor who has not developed the professional maturity to tolerate intractable illness characterized by setbacks is apt to blame the patient for the doctor's own sense of failure. This is inexcusable. There is no benefit to either physician or patient in viewing chronic illness as a struggle that must be won. The real issue is how to maximize the patient's comfort and productivity. In the doctor-patient relationship, neither doctor nor patient "owes" recovery to the other. What both do owe each other is respectful, attentive, and responsive behavior. This is a good formula for strengthening the medical partnership.

In any situation typified by uncertainty, the mind will attempt to fill in the information deficit as well as it can. Very strong feelings are the most likely ones to be projected onto the blank screen of the unknown. Thus, Paul Adams reexperienced old guilt associated with Karen's heart murmur. As the reader knows, there is no objective reason to feel guilty. It was not his fault. Parents always experience some guilt if a child has a constitutional weakness. The guilt is powerful, irrational, and often not conscious. In the face of uncertainty, Bill was beginning to be fearful and angry. He stopped himself from fully experiencing these emotions because they made him feel helpless. He filled the space left by uncertainty by keeping himself busy. Karen's projected feeling was fear that she was going to die, or be seriously ill (unable to heal) for the foreseeable future.

That uncertainty is highly stressful cannot be disputed. Even dogs when presented by Pavlov with ambiguous stimuli felt severe stress. People are more resourceful than dogs, however. They can ask for clarification and tolerate uncertainty if they understand that at some point there will be light at the end of the tunnel. It is wise to be aware of the emotional drain uncertainty creates so that one can diminish the anxiety before it becomes intolerable. People assuage anxiety in different ways: time with a friend, an entertaining book to read, the counsel of a minister or therapist.

Major life changes may cause one to swing from psychological denial of the new reality to a sense of being overwhelmed by it. Major life transitions such as changes in health, marital, or financial status, or even significant birthdays, are events that are difficult to incorporate into one's self-definition. A new event is likely to trigger simultaneously a longing for the past and a keen awareness of the present. Since transitions are apt to bring with them heightened anxiety, people often react by denying to themselves that any change has really occurred; at other times they may feel overpowered by the change. Until the new event with its accompanying fear has been incorporated into an expanded view of oneself, there is little middle ground of realistic thought or action.

Bill is a little less resilient than either Karen or Paul, and thus he was able to experience consciously only one end of the spectrum, namely, the denial of any real change. This is indicated by his belief that the doctors would "fix" Karen. All other possibilities he kept from awareness. Reality, of course, offers no guarantees, and a person like Bill is ill-equipped to deal with the news that a loved one is not going to be "fixed" if that should be the eventual medical outcome.

Bill's fear of an altered future is so powerful that he cannot even explore in fantasy the possibility of change due to illness This is not optimism, but a sign that Bill is not adequately tracking reality. Karen is very ill, and it would be helpful to Bill if he could explore, at least in his thoughts, what would be required of him if Karen's recovery is slow or nonexistent. If he does not need to pretend that the facts about Karen are different from the reality, he will more quickly be able to settle into dealing competently with the here and now. Focusing attention on the present, without getting trapped in either the past or the future, permits optimism, courage, and dogged determination to deal with things as they are.

The emotions imposed by illness often produce a sense of being absolutely alone. It is as if no one could possibly understand or empathize with the stark emotions being felt by the patient and his family. Paul Adams temporarily experiences a sense of isolation when he perceives the hospital environment as divided into "them" and "us," with the "us" being isolated individuals in a hospital bed or waiting room. Some of the anger inherent in this perception is abated when he accepts Miss Smith's invitation to be sociable in the waiting room.

A sense of being alone may take the form of not recognizing or accepting sources of help or comfort. Bill experiences this to some extent in his attempts to cope with the crisis without using the supports available to him to their maximum. In its extreme form, this tactic leads to self-martyrdom, which may be borne in sullen silence or with ungracious outbreaks of fury.

Emotional isolation in the lives of some people may be encountered for the very first time when illness strikes. Karen seems to have a group of friends from work who are eager to let their presence and support be known. We can speculate that in many ways, Karen is not alone. Yet, for all of us, there are some encounters with fate whose primary emotional impact is a solitary one. There is no way to deny that one is seriously ill. One is aware of the many organic functions that no longer operate with smooth harmony. This is truly a shocking and lonely awareness. Karen knows she is in fragile physical condition. She is afraid because she does not know what will happen, and death seems all too close at hand. The initial awareness that one is only mortal, and that the body can fail in serious ways, is a shock. One feels that this powerful awareness cannot be shared by others, but this is not true. We are all mortal, and emotional reaction to illness can be shared, and in the sharing some of the pain and fear can be alleviated. There is a critical role in the life of the chronically ill person to be filled by family, friends, and medical personnel. Frequently, life for the patient becomes intolerable at the point where it seems family and friends are withdrawing from him. It is crucial that this perception be examined very carefully to determine if it is valid. It may be that the patient simply does not know how to ask for all the help he needs. It may be that the family and friends will not or cannot provide adequate support. In either case the patient is experiencing profound deprivation.

We will look at emotional isolation in more detail in the next chapter.

CHAPTER TWO

ISOLATION

The rain hung heavily in the air before it finally began to fall with soft splattering sounds. Evie Barnat was relieved to finally be able to hear the sound of late winter and to sense the denseness of the gray clouds. She was comfortably seated in a rocker with a cup of steaming tea held loosely in her hand, a morning ritual that in recent months had stretched to consume most of the day. Sitting, rocking, thinking, feeling. Maybe in an hour or so she could think of someone to call by dreaming up an excuse to hear another's voice. Her husband would not be home until dinner, and it was not even lunch time yet.

Evie had developed juvenile diabetes when she was ten. She had been frightened by her illness initially, but later, when she saw the devastation on her parents' faces, she became terrified. After she had spent some time in the hospital, the doctors ascertained what the problem was. Her parents began reading furiously about juvenile diabetes. The more they read, the sadder and more anxious they became. She had learned to give herself injections and had changed her diet; and then she also began to look at some of the journal articles about diabetes. It seemed awful but unreal to her.

The articles said terrible things could happen in adulthood—circulatory, visual, and kidney failures. She, however, would just go on with her life—none of that would happen to her.

Over the years, Evie's health remained stable. She had a variety of insulin reactions when the dosage was not quite right for her state of nutrition and level of exercise. She had one or two blackouts and awoke in the college health center. For the most part, however, she just did not let herself think about her illness. She took care of herself most of the time and tried to show her parents, friends, and, later, her husband that she was just fine.

She began seeing Jack, her husband-to-be, while she was in college. He was ten years her senior, and they had met by chance in a bookstore. She was a major in graphic arts. Jack was an electrician. He'd interested her then, as now, because he was intense, self-sufficient, unhampered by his family's exhortations to "do something" with his intellect that would lead to his making large sums of money.

She had told him soon after they began dating about her diabetes, and he seemed to take it in stride. She could not help wondering where he had hidden the anxiety and disappointment she'd expected her disclosure to create. She was 22 and he 32 when they married. They lived modestly, but comfortably, on his salary and her freelancing as a graphic artist. The idea of adding children to the family was never really discussed, and they seemed content to be a family of two with very active social lives and enough hard work to fill most days.

Life had changed abruptly one day when she was laying out a series of logo designs for a new customer. Her vision seemed cloudy, and she was having trouble seeing the lower field of vision. Since her night vision was also becoming steadily worse, she consulted an opthamologist. He confirmed one of her worst fears. The diabetes had begun to affect her eyes. Before she had a chance to ask even a few questions, the doctor had her scheduled for laser treatments. The nurse told her to have her husband bring her to the clinic the next morning. She was not told that the treatments were painful or that even if they were successful in staunching the hemorrhage in one place, it was possible other blood vessels would have to be treated in the future.

Her husband was wonderful. He never complained about the interruptions to his life, and he held her close when her fear became unbearable. But they never really talked about the personal fears either one of them was feeling. All the words of emotional distress were silenced. Looking back at the abrupt changes in their lives that illness had wrought, Evie felt they had managed well with the uncertainty and the trauma of the treatments. On another level, though, she was beginning to feel disquieted.

In the beginning, Evie had been very hopeful that the treatments would work. They certainly helped, but the hemorrhaging was much more widespread than was thought at first. Many, many treatments with periods of respite between them—they seemed to fill her whole life. She had turned her customers over to a friend until she could return to work. The pleasant social interruptions to her workday had also become a thing of the past. She could not drive—she hoped this was temporary—and she was housebound. She hated to ask friends to leave work, pick her up for lunch, and return her home. It seemed like a real imposition.

She tried to stay in touch by phone. She called friends, relatives, her modern dance instructor to explain her absence from class; she called the March of Dimes to decline their request that she be fundraising chairman for her block—she called anyone she could think of. Maybe two hours of calls a day. That became her work—just trying to stay in touch.

One day she put the phone down in the middle of dialing her best friend. She had nothing to say that this friend hadn't heard ten times already. She felt alone and terrified. Outside it was still the lightest, brightest part of the day. She usually did not become terrified until the sun began to go down and the light lost its intensity. By late afternoon, she had all the lights in the house on so that she could continue to move about freely. With each light she turned on, though, she wondered how long it would be before she really was blind. She had no defense against this fear, and she hated to burden her husband with it. He was beginning to look tired. The loss of her income along with the increase in medical expenses was wearing on him. Or maybe it was all the extra considerations, the little things he did to be helpful to her, the willingness to tackle the housework on days she was recovering from a treatment. She wasn't supposed to lift things anymore. Her husband did the shopping, put the iron skillets on the stove for her, and did the laundry. The more work he did, the less they made love. The less physical contact they had, the more they seemed like polite strangers sharing a house. During the day, she cried for reasons to which she could give no easy words. During the night, he worried and felt inadequate.

More and more often Evie withdrew to her rocker with a cup of tea to look out the window and see what she could still see. She played games with herself. How much of that painting can I see from ten paces today? These checking-up games became compulsive rituals, and she felt she was crumbling a little more inside each time she discerned that she was seeing less.

Her life seemed divided into two segments: before and after. Before and after what, exactly, was unclear. Before included all the time she was working, enjoying her friends, and taking care of her husband. After began with her vision problem, but where it would end was distressingly unclear. Before was a life with a great deal of social contact. After was a string of phone calls she made to friends who seemed distant. Not quite cold, but distant and unaware. They tried to tell her how bad the flu was that went around town last week. Why couldn't they listen to how awful it was to know her body was terribly vulnerable? She didn't want to know who won the bridge tournament. She wanted someone to hold her hand, cry with her, make her tea and cookies. These were the thoughts occupying Evie during most of each unbearably long day, and intruding into her sleep, causing nightmares and restlessness.

Evie felt her illness had made her a nonperson. Okay. She was going to be the best nonperson she knew how to be. No demands on anyone. No requests for assistance. No more telephone calls to friends who did not call back or who called and hastily apologized for their long lack of contact, their too-busy lives. Yes. Their lives were too busy for a friend who could no longer be a recreation partner.

Evie did not understand how much of her decision to launch a cold war on her friends and family was based on her anger. She just felt relieved from some of her fear by making a clear choice to withdraw. For the duration of the day she was able to think of herself. She thought about all that she had lost—all the changes in her once-satisfying life that had been made against her will by a body that would not function as it once had. She thought of her career and how that was lost to her if she in fact became blind. The sadness in these thoughts outweighed her fear, and she cried her way through the lunch hour.

Evie cried and the rain continued. By three that afternoon it was necessary to switch on all the lights in the living room. It was no comfort that she would have had to turn on most of them simply because it was raining, even if her eyes were not a problem. The need for artificial light was now a direct blow to her self-esteem. She had to turn the light on to brighten her field of vision, even during the day—hence she judged herself defective. She felt almost numb walking around the room turning on lamps. Numb was a pretty good word for how she felt most of the time. The numbness disguised the sadness, making it less painful and less real. She passed day after day in numb defiance of her illness, her disability, and her separation from friends.

By four, Evie began thinking about dinner. Jack would be home by 5:30. They would watch the news and then eat at seven. She tried to plan meals that would require her presence in the kitchen until the news came on. That way she would not feel she was in Jack's way. He would not have to notice that she was wandering around in a daze, and she could feel productively busy for the first time during the entire day. When she was first receiving laser treatments, the two of them had talked a lot about how she was doing. They both felt somewhat optimistic and decisive. Active people, they were taking action and life would improve. Now Evie wasn't at all sure. The treatments had been going on for two months; she was due for a checkup at the end of the week. She no longer could judge if her eyes were the same or clearing. She was worried about the appointment and did not want to face the possibility that further treatments would be prescribed. She was tired, and alone.

Having stopped to buy a bouquet of flowers, Jack was a few minutes late getting home. When Evie saw him a spark of her non-numb self reappeared. He looked comical wrestling with the door, the flowers, and the dog who leapt to meet him.

"They are beautiful. What are they for?"

Jack kissed her hello briefly and smiled. "I thought we needed to celebrate the raise I just got today." Evie could see he was very proud of his surprise news. Half of her wanted to react in her customary, demonstrative style. But these were not customary days, and she felt the numbness take hold again. She was genuinely pleased for him, but any news of his job seemed to make her feel all the more useless. So she congratulated him quietly and returned to the kitchen.

"I thought it would make you happy. I don't seem to be able to do anything right."

Evie, aware of Jack's anger, began to cry. "It's my fault, I'm sorry I just feel so terribly alone that I sometimes forget we are struggling together."

Jack closed his arms around her, and she felt somewhat better. They ate early, in front of the TV. Jack had been invited out bowling with friends of theirs.

"Why don't you come. You'll feel better if you're not here alone."

"I haven't talked to the Craemers for months. I wouldn't have anything to tell them."

Jack responded, "Have it your way. I know they would like to see you. You really seem determined to make it hard on yourself."

"It's not my way, my decision. Susan could have called me back just once after all the times I've left messages for her. I did not hear one word from her. I would feel funny going tonight and pretending everything is just fine."

"Why don't you go and let her know everything is not all right?" Jack and Evie began to laugh. The idea of Evie sticking up for herself was so outrageous it was almost comical. She had never been able to risk the possibility of rejection by stating her views directly.

"I think I will just stay home."

"Suit yourself," Jack replied. He gathered up his bowling gear quickly and shut the door noisily behind him.

Evie loaded the dishwasher and then sank into her rocker. She was trying to decide whether she should watch TV or listen to music when the telephone rang.

"Evie?"

"Yes."

"It's Stephanie. Am I interrupting anything?"

"Of course not. Jack's out bowling, and I'm here feeling sorry for myself."

"Good. Then you won't mind if I come over. I've got hot gingerbread and a couple of casseroles to put in your freezer."

"That's really nice, Stephanie, but I don't want you to go to the trouble."

"Nonsense, Evie. The gingerbread is getting cold. Now just put on the teakettle and I'll be over in ten minutes."

Stephanie was an enigma. She and Evie had briefly worked together for a company the previous year. Then Evie began freelancing and Stephanie stayed on in the firm. They saw each other infrequently in the course of business—usually at the printer's. Their relationship was cordial, but not close. When Evie became ill, Stephanie began calling regularly to say hello. Evie always felt a little funny about the fact that Stephanie, and not her close friends, was the one who knew the most about her physical condition. Stephanie did not seem put off. She did not act frightened, and she did not make Evie feel like a charity case. She did make Evie feel inadequate, though. How was she ever going to repay Stephanie's kindness? When Evie raised this issue, Stephanie dismissed it. People need help sometimes was all she had said. But Evie wondered if she really needed this much help. She could still cook. It wasn't a wake, after all. On the other hand, it made her feel cared for to have a friend willing to invest time in her welfare.

The evening passed very quickly. They ate the gingerbread—made according to a recipe for diabetics—with gusto and laughed their way through several cups of tea. Stephanie had a wonderful way of including Evie in the goings-on at work without making her feel unproductive. She asked Evie's advice on design problems, and told her about the antics of the printer's assistant.

When Jack returned, Stephanie questioned him closely about his game and included him effortlessly into the pleasantness the women had been sharing. Jack liked her very much and responded to her vivaciousness and intensity. She reminded him of Evie before Evie had become so preoccupied.

The Barnats said goodnight to their guest. Immediately, a tension that had been absent between them in Stephanie's presence returned. They avoided it for a time by locking doors and turning off lights. Then, they walked arm in arm, deliberately, almost shyly, to their room.

COMMENTARY

As is often the case, Evie and Jack weathered the acute episode of Evie's illness well. Neither one succumbed to panic, and they were able to maintain a primarily positive attitude toward one another. Evie was supported through the laser treatments by Jack, who demonstrated his caring and concern by being helpful to Evie through his actions, rather than through words. To their later detriment, however, they did not talk much about their anxieties, focusing instead entirely on the treatment. During a crisis episode, action is extremely important, but in the later stages of emotional transition created by illness, it is not sufficient. The patient's resiliency and emotional outlook is greatly enhanced by a supportive talking relationship with family, friends, doctors, and, if desired, counselors.

To free both patient and family from isolation, all those involved must be able to talk to each other directly about their painful and frightening feelings. In the case of Evie and Jack, talking through their feelings was not a strong point in their marriage. Perhaps both were somewhat passive about their opinions, shy about their feelings, or simply afraid of taking risks. It is significant, for example, that this couple took no active role in deciding whether or not to have a family. It was a topic that was simply not discussed. Clues about how well a couple can do with the emotionally charged issues of illness can often be obtained by looking at what the customary pattern has been in communicating about other emotionally meaningful or difficult issues. The clue that having children was too hot a topic to be discussed suggests that other important issues involving the couple will likewise be avoided. In the case of illness, part of the reason for not talking about the individual feelings of the marriage partners involved is the rather magical thought that if something is not discussed, it is not real. Illness can often be denied conscious, intellectual reality, even while it is completely dominating one's life. We see that in this case. Neither husband nor wife expresses their feelings of disappointment, despair, anger, or fear, so as not to burden the other one or frighten oneself. Clearly, expressing painful feelings is difficult, and sometimes the right words seem to be lacking; but isn't the price of denying reality by silence too high? What is silent can grow more frightening and distorted than what is spoken. Evie and Jack both feel inadequate, and unworthy. They have stopped speaking at all to one another with ease. Their tempers are short because of the strain they are under. Even in their intimate life, neither feels secure with the other. Their zest for one another returns in Stephanie's company when each can focus on a high quality interchange and not on the lack of communication.

The emptiness and loneliness experienced so graphically by Evie has its counterpart in Jack. Chronic illness is a family problem and is not confined to the ill member. Under the best of circumstances, family dynamics are complex. With illness to further obscure the means by which a family functions productively, it can be very easy to lose sight of the goal that most families strive for: to be responsively and respectfully aware of other family members.

Evie mistakenly believes that she is taking care of Jack by forcing him out of her life and not talking to him about her worries. Over time, she made the same error with her friends. The error was in deciding for Jack and for her friends that she was simply a burden and had nothing to offer anyone other than a tale of woe. The more she convinced herself of this, the less she had to offer. Evie's growing self-martyrdom is a complicated issue, however, because it has some justification. She was deeply hurt by friends who could not make time for her in their lives—not even for a phone call. There are several issues involved here.

Illness temporarily disrupts the social support network of the patient and family. The more casual and less personal the contacts, the more easily they are disrupted. Superficial relationships are the first to be lost. A corollary of this is that the more a relationship is based on only one shared purpose, idea, or value, the easier it is for the relationship to become disrupted. Evie felt entirely abandoned by her friends at work. Apparently, these friendships were based primarily on working closely together in the same environment. When Evie could not participate at work, she felt there was no friendship. In part, her work friends may have retreated from her due to their own discomfort concerning illness, but to the extent that it occurred, their separation was aided and abetted by Evie's feeling that she could not be direct with her friends and ask for support. In most cases, it is a combination of the vulnerability of both friends and patient that seems to result in the very commonly experienced distance between people who previously had been part of each other's daily lives. If Evie and her work friends had had other sources of compatibility beyond the coincidence of working together, there would have been other ties helping the relationships to remain functional.

Opportunities for contact sometimes are avoided because of anger and fear. The recreational-social outlets of couples are almost always badly disrupted for a time. This is especially devastating because the spouse needs a way to keep emotionally replenished in order to remain of assistance to the patient and to maintain his own well-being. It is a healthy sign that Jack continued his bowling alliance with the Craemers. It would have been even more encouraging if Evie could have let herself go along and keep the group company. She could not have played, but she would have been supporting Jack in his attempt to retain continuity in their lives. A problem for Evie was that her anger might demand expression. She might have had to speak her mind to her friend and thus risk rejection, something she greatly feared. The primary difficulty in Evie's case is that she has always had a limited view of what relationships consist of. From childhood on, she felt she could only be valuable to the people who knew her by denying her illness and pretending all was well all of the time. At the current time, little is well, and she is at a complete loss to experience herself as having a meaningful and viable life that can be shared with others.

In one regard, however, Evie is more fortunate than some chronically ill people. Even though Jack feels he has lost the ability to please her, he does try to maintain a close relationship with Evie. So does Stephanie, in the face of little encouragement from Evie. There are cases, however, where the patient has had friendships based on shared values and experiences, understands that part of friendship is to be available when needed, feels that he has done this well for others, and still is confronted by a social vacuum following illness. When this occurs, the patient experiences tremendous despair and self-doubt.

The most common complaint among the chronically ill is that friends whom they have relied on for many years abruptly abandon them when they become ill. This complaint exists among all types of people—martyrs and nonmartyrs, friendly and surly, of all socioeconomic levels. It is searing testimony of one of the greatest sadnesses of chronic illness. It will not change the reality, but it may help to understand that this type of emotional abandonment is the product of fear. Seeing the devastation of illness in a loved one reminds the observer that his time, too, will come. No one is immune to the possibility of bodily failure. It is unfortunate, as well as astonishing, that our culture makes it so difficult to accept the inevitable.

There are communities where illness does not lead to rejection, where life is seen as a process that does not become worthless just because one has become ill. These communities, almost by definition, are less transient than ours, and have ties that extend beyond shared interests in recreation or employment. Notable among these groups for its way of dealing with illness and death are the Amish.

Over a period of years, however, the patient usually figures out which friends are especially missed and why. He then begins the process of reclaiming those who are reclaimable by making the overtures and taking the initiative in contacting these friends, who may be paralyzed by their feeling of inadequacy and helplessness to help someone they love.

The relationships that do endure through an illness may not be the ones expected. Evie was surprised and puzzled that her relationship with Stephanie endured while closer ones were disrupted. She was quite amazed at Stephanie's easy and continuous giving of herself, even though the two women had not been particularly close at work. In this relationship, we cannot underestimate Stephanie's resilience in the face of anxiety. She seems to be the kind of person that is able to perceive a need and then act to relieve it. Somewhere in her background she was well enough cared for and nurtured that it is not overwhelming for her to give of herself and care for another in need.

There is an important difference between healthy caring for and unhealthy care taking. The concept that doing for another is rewarding in and of itself, which is so clearly developed in Stephanie, is not much developed in Evie's personality; much more prominent is her need to make everyone feel that she is physically fine, that she will never be a burden.

As a child, Evie responded to her illness responsibly by learning what she needed to do for herself and then doing it. So far so good. But she must have felt great concern about the fear her parents demonstrated about her diabetes. To some extent, she felt she had brought trouble to her parents and that she would have to dispel it. She began to minimize her concerns about her illness as a way of comforting her family and friends. To alleviate their guilt and fear, as well as her own, she would be "normal," no trouble to anyone. Thus her history of denying, or hiding, her actual physical condition and her fears concerning it began very early. Almost certainly, her efforts to be like all the other children were rewarded by family and friends. To some extent, it was good for her not to assume she was completely different from other children; however, by making her diabetes a secret, she did not have the chance to discover that her personality and the way she treated other people were at the core of how people responded to her—not her physical status.

Evie's awareness of the feelings of others and her attempts to make them happy were the action of an appealing young girl. As a child, she could not understand that one human being cannot be entirely responsible for another's well-being. As an adult, she continued trying to make herself solely responsible for everyone else's feelings. This sense of responsibility mistakenly equates management of other people's feelings (an impossible task) with caring for them. Apparently, Evie felt she could be socially desirable only if she could "protect" the feelings of other people by keeping them distanced from her illness. Contrast this with the healthy "caring for" other people that is evidenced by Stephanie. Evie is trapped by her misconception and poor self-esteem. She has judged herself harshly without allowing her friends to tell her that she was not a burden. The less contact with social reality Evie had, the more compelling was her feeling that she was a failure—a flawed, unlovable woman. This burden of sadness is more than anyone should be required to bear alone.

A closely related issue is the question, How much should a patient do for himself and how much should he lean on others for help and support? By saying that the burden of sadness created by illness is not one that need be borne alone, I do not mean to imply that the patient should cease taking responsibility for himself. It is necessary for his self-esteem—as well as for family harmony—that the patient be enterprising in attempting to solve problems, but this need not be done in isolation. In Evie's situation, a very dependent person would be making an endless string of demands disguised as requests of Jack. Even with severe vision problems, it is possible for a person to become quite independent. This might require special mobility training with a cane, learning the bus system, and reorganizing the house so that items in frequent use are readily available and not lost in jumbled drawers. It will require special consideration from other members of the household to see that objects are always returned to the same place after use and no hazards are left on the floor for the visually impaired person to trip on.

It is often useful for the patient to learn something of his illness and its management. Information gathering—if it reduces anxiety—may take the form of an extra appointment with the doctor, independent reading, or of consulting an organization, such as the local county diabetes association.* These are all active steps either taken alone by the ill member of the family or in conjunction with another family member.

Just as it is necessary for the patient to keep trying in order to feel worthwhile, it is necessary to ask for help when confronted with tasks that cannot or should not be accomplished alone. An example in Evie's case was lifting cast-iron pans to the range. Help may be solicited in the more general form of requests for support from friends. Good, solid contact is needed, that lets the patient confide his feelings or allows the patient to be distracted from his physical woes by hearing the local gossip or catching up on activity in an area

---

*Not all people will feel less anxious by receiving more information. For some, anticipating further decline in their health on the basis of what can be statistically expected can lead to a morbid preoccupation with symptoms that may never occur in their own cases. For others, having as much information as possible about the course of their illness gives them a sense of preparation and control over circumstances, and might allow early recognition of important physiological changes which could aid treatment. There is no one correct response to this choice of knowing or not knowing.

of interest. The friend who is blessed with a sense of humor and sends cartoons or tells amusing stories is a real prize.

It may take a long time for the patient to learn how to ask for help appropriately. Requests for assistance should not be so frequent that they represent all the traffic can bear. If this is done, the social support network dries up, leaving the patient without helpers. Nor should requests be so minimal that they give everyone the idea that an offer of help would be seen as an insult. The requests should be made on the basis of need. A need exists if the patient feels physically or emotionally unable to manage alone. A need does not exist if the requests are really an attempt to control other people, and are not in genuine response to a need imposed by the illness or other circumstances.

These are tricky waters to navigate, and most families flounder occasionally. If the floundering is not self-correcting through family discussion, and the failure to appreciate the needs of others becomes a chronic condition, then family therapy may be in order. Counseling can be very useful in breaking up the logjams of old, nonfunctional patterns of relating that we all experience.

The single person who is without benefit of support from family and who has few friends is especially at risk during the isolation phase. Already socially isolated, this individual needs to show great perseverance in locating social services available. Even the tedious and sometimes frustrating job of looking through the phone book for social services is an important beginning. One contact leads to another and becomes the way of developing a productive network of support. Some patients have found it useful to become involved themselves as helpers of others who are suffering. In this way they achieve their goal of enhanced social contact, and have a chance to be reminded of some of their own qualities that are separate from the disease.

An important thing to remember: *Asking for help may be the most effective way to guarantee true independence and control in a life that is subjected to the limitations imposed by illness.* Evie does not have a very mature concept of friendship yet, so she does not understand that in healthy friendships, friends take care of one another. Her life could be enriched far beyond sitting in a rocker drinking tea alone. Her incredibly powerful reluctance to ask a friend to pick her up for a lunch date or come over to gossip makes her life much more limited than it has to be. Independence suggests being able to choose options. One choice is to ask a friend to provide companionship, but far too few people consider such action independent. In part, this is because society has perpetuated a myth that the chronically ill are unreasonably demanding and apt to feel sorry for themselves. While it is an accurate picture of some individuals already characterized by anger and extreme dependence, it certainly is not an inherent part of the picture of chronic illness. People having such personality problems will bring these problems to their illness; people with more resilient, resourceful personalities will show evidence of these healthier traits in the situation of illness.

There are other reasons why it is difficult to ask for help. If one has been reared to be fiercely self-sufficient, for instance, it may not even cross the patient's mind to ask another "to inconvenience himself." However, the primary reason for difficulty in asking for help is guilt feelings about having an illness. This is true of Evie. This sort of guilt can be extremely destructive of the patient's self-esteem by causing the patient to remain secluded when the need for companionship is very high. Manifestations of such guilt need to be watched carefully. Patients like Evie do very well in psychotherapy, becoming progressively more able to accept themselves and receive the acceptance of others.

There is one final point in Evie's case that needs fuller discussion because it often occurs as a reaction to the abandonment patients feel as their isolation and introspection deepen. Evie decided not only not to bother family and friends with her feelings, but also to adopt the posture of being the best nonperson she could be. In other words, she felt that if she, the person with physical problems, was not going to be valued by the people she cared about, then she, the vulnerable and frightened person, would simply cease to exist as an entity to reckon with. Evie was ready to consign herself to the status of one with no needs and no relationships to others because she was angry and hurt. She felt that others saw her as she saw herself—a person who is flawed and who must, therefore, be cast on the scrap heap. It is very important that this kind of anger be recognized as self-destructive. Evie was voluntarily cutting herself off emotionally from potential sources of assistance. True, many of her friends had disappointed her. And she really had tried very hard to maintain contact with people that she no longer saw on a daily basis. But the leap from feeling rejected by some friends, who were probably paralyzed by their own weaknesses and not by Evie's illness, to wanting to resign from the human race is a very large one and cannot be dismissed lightly. It suggests that Evie is given to self-torment and that her emotional reconstitution and adaptation to her illness will be slow and hard.

Evie seems given to self-doubt and self-blame. She has temporarily lost contact with what she likes in herself. People like Evie spend a great deal of time in the isolation stage, continuing to withdraw and accepting nothing from others, however freely given. It is probably more accurate to say that they feel so impoverished by the stress exacted by their physical plight that they accept little and give less and less to those who are there to support them. The stage is set for the accumulation of extreme psychic pain.

Because Evie consciously recognizes she has supporters and allies, she will not be able to convert this pain to anger for some time. The pain is already so intense that she finds it preferable to impose psychological numbness on herself rather than experience its strength. How, then, would she deal with anger? Anger risks giving offense to those sources of support available to her—sources that Evie sees as frail and diminishing. Further, anger is in no way consistent with Evie's conception of what makes her socially desirable, and thus her own overt anger would be very frightening to her. Again numbness seems preferable. This choice is rarely a fully conscious one, and it springs from the depths of a person's self-protective instincts. As a child Evie had found it useful to maintain her social desirability by disguising the fact that she had a serious medical condition. As an adult, her symptoms are more noticeable to others, and she is trying so hard to mask them—and her emotional turmoil—that she presents a stony, unemotional surface rather than to feel she is requiring others to be aware of her distress. The mask is only a surface distortion of very powerful feelings, and it is more than likely that Evie is the only one who is fooled by the masquerade.

Emotional numbness is a state that can come about solely as a reaction against the grief engendered by illness, or it may be induced through chemical means by alcohol or drugs. Therefore, it is sometimes discovered that sleeping or pain medication is being abused or that the patient has dramatically increased his alcohol consumption. In either case, it is an attempt by the patient to dull savage surges of anxiety, grief, or rage.

When a patient is more aware of his feelings than Evie is, the sadness associated with isolation causes a swifter transition from an introspective awareness of loss to a multilevel expression of anger. That is, the pain of losing a concept of oneself as a healthy and productive person combines with estrangement from friends and family to create rage. In the chronically ill patient, fear and sadness, the emotions most typical of the crisis and isolation phases, are often experienced before rage. Some people, however, begin by having to deal with rage as their preliminary emotional step toward regaining a sense of emotional wholeness. The experiences described in the next chapter are not unusual, even though they are much more graphic in the case I present than in some others.

CHAPTER THREE

ANGER

Edward stood up and wanted to scream. Where was the floor and where was he in relation to it? He widened his stance hoping that would ease the sense of vertigo and stabilize his balance. It helped some, and he felt able to try a few steps. Because his balance was so poor, he walked with a rocking motion rather than with clear forward progress, shifting his weight from one of his widely spaced feet to the other.

He managed the 15 steps to the bathroom with considerable difficulty, and leaned heavily against the washstand for support. Edward was completely exhausted—wide awake, but exhausted. It was already four a.m. and he had been up for two hours, hoping in vain to be able to return to sleep. Sleeping these days was no longer the simple, natural state it had been six months ago. He was barely able to sleep, and when he did he was troubled by vivid nightmares so closely paralleling reality that there was little rest in the hours of sleep.

Edward was only 48, at the peak of a productive career in petroleum products research. He was accustomed to using his intelligence to overcome almost any difficulty. Problems were not usually stacked up like airplanes over a crowded airport. Now he had them in spades, and even though Edward was not a weak man, he was tiring with the effort to assign them proper priorities. Difficulties he could not resolve began when his 22-year marriage ended in divorce three years earlier. And just when he was getting back on his feet emotionally and socially, an old physical problem flared up, destroying any semblance of tranquility he had achieved since his divorce.

For many years, Edward had known that he had multiple sclerosis (MS), a little-understood disorder of the central nervous system. In his case, its earliest symptoms had been relatively minor—weakness in one leg, a disruption of his fine motor coordination, making it difficult to write at times, and strange prickly sensations on the skin of his legs. None of these symptoms had been permanent, and since he was primarily bothered by fatigue, he treated his own case by going to bed as if he had a cold until he felt somewhat better. Later, more troubling symptoms developed, including numbness and difficulty in walking due to extreme weakness.

Until this last episode, he never had to take off more than a week from work before. Since the treatment of MS is as individual as the manifestations of the disease, and since very little exists in the way of effective treatment, Edward had not been treated with medication until recently. But this episode was much more serious than any he had previously encountered, and the neurologist, whom he trusted and liked, put Edward on very high doses of steroids. These drugs reduce inflammation, it is thought, and shorten a severe episode. The drugs were powerful ones indeed, and his doctor was very good about informing Edward of some of the side effects so that he would not be too alarmed if they began to occur. When the disease process showed no signs of lessening in its intensity, his neurologist raised the already high dose of medication. Soon after—and the doctor told Edward he was not sure if it was due to the medication or if the disease had run out of steam for a while—the daily losses of sensation and motor function began to level off. Edward had become very frightened by the extremely swift loss of function, and was greatly relieved when he could wake up in the morning and find that nothing more was lost during the time he slept. He had been out of work for six months, and his strength was just now beginning to return. Even so, a trip to the bathroom, walking unsupported by a cane or walker, required every ounce of strength he possessed. He wondered if he would ever play handball again.

Since his divorce, Edward had become quite independent, and he kept a pleasant apartment with a sunny view of the hills. He had a housekeeper in once a week, but he had learned to fend for himself the days she did not work for him. He found he enjoyed knowing everything was shipshape and just the way he liked it. When he had become ill, he could not care for himself at all, and the doctor had given him a choice: he could check into the hospital so that he would be assured of attention if he needed it, or he could hire a home nurse to look after him, prepare meals, check that he took his medications, and get him to the doctor if necessary.

Edward hated dependence and had inwardly rebelled at the idea, even though he knew he could not take care of himself. He had never asked anything of anyone, he told himself, and now he had no choice but to go to the hospital if he could not bring himself to ask for assistance. As seeking help seemed the lesser of two evils, he did hire a daytime nurse and arranged for a friend or one of his children to come by after dinner to see that he was set for the night. He thought he was an efficient man when it came to detail, until he tried to work out a schedule for the people who were to look after him. Now that he was somewhat stronger, he did not need quite so much help, so the nurse and the son with the most free time were easily able to satisfy Edward's requirements.

From the day he had begun taking steroids, Edward noticed he was having great trouble sleeping. He was fitful, and often could not sleep until he was on the brink of physical exhaustion. His mind was spinning with a thousand thoughts at once, yet time seemed to go by in painful slowness. He was worried about a great many things. He would begin worrying about when he could return to work, say, and soon find himself worrying about whether his savings account was in the bank paying the highest interest. He reported his difficulty sleeping to the doctor, who, although concerned, told him that it was a common reaction to the medication.

Then Edward began feeling blue. He felt keenly the loss of managing at an efficient level. He was used to being a very thorough man—a careful researcher, meticulous, and organized. His life now seemed so helter-skelter, just a matter of getting from one hour to the next without calamity. These thoughts made Edward sad, but worse than sad, they made him feel completely powerless to affect his destiny in a satisfactory way. He was sick of being sick, and tired of waiting for his fatigue to lift and some of his old energy to reappear. He felt completely worthless, as if all he had worked so gladly to attain in his life was gone for good. Some of these feelings were like ones he remembered when he was desperately lonely following his divorce. After his divorce, he felt like part of his life had died, but this time he felt like he had died. It was a miserable joke that, in fact, he continued to live. It's a cowardly disease, he thought, one that can maim, but usually does not kill.

Edward's mood became progressively sadder. He told himself that he had good reason for his depression, but somehow his blue feelings went beyond his physical problems. He had a terrible sense of being mired down in this sadness, as if emotionally he were trying to move through glue and could not do it. He also felt as if he were trying to move through glue physically. Sometimes he could not keep one foot from dragging slightly as he walked. He was feeling more desperate than he ever had in his entire life; he was in a panic on the inside, without being able to do anything in the outside world to help himself feel better and less afraid. He was afraid now, not just in a physical sense, but because he did not recognize the emotions of the man staring at him in the mirror. He felt so sad that he wanted to cry, and at the same time he wanted to giggle like a maniac. People told him he was talking very fast—when he talked at all—and he could go for days carrying on conversations just inside his head.

Even his doctor noticed a change. He told Edward that since the illness seemed to be abating, and Edward was beginning to feel some of the harmful side effects of the medication, they would need to begin withdrawing the drug. When Edward asked if he couldn't simply stop taking the medication, his doctor was firm; with drugs this powerful, he said, a careful, medically determined schedule using Edward's subjective reports of the withdrawal experience would be necessary.

Today was to be the first day of gradual withdrawal from medication. Edward had written the schedule out carefully and taped it to the medicine chest so that he would not get confused. It seemed that he did get confused easily these days, and that he sometimes forgot the simplest bits of information. He was not going to forget these important instructions, though, and he reread them carefully.

Abruptly, something caught his attention from the corner of his eye. He couldn't really see it clearly, but something was being reflected by the mirror. He wearily wiped his eyes, scanned the bathroom for an insect that might have caused his attention to flicker from the prescription paper he was reading. He spotted nothing and returned to reviewing the instructions for the day. Picking up his comb, he absently began tidying the hair framing his puffy, bloated face. It was not possible to discern the familiar, angular jaw and cheekbones because they were obscured by the medication-induced fluid retention from which he now suffered. He absolutely hated the way he looked, and the additional 30 pounds of weight he carried dragged at him with every lumbering motion he made. It was bad enough that he might never walk easily again, but did he have to look so awful at the same time? He began feeling very angry, silently cursing the disease, fate, medicine for not having any useful answers, and most of all his own bodily weakness that made it possible for a disease to take over his life. He knew no one with this illness, and most of the time he felt like a freak who knew what he wanted to do but who could not get his muscles to respond to his wishes.

Edward ran a hand over the stubble of his beard and decided not to shave. This was odd: even when he was very ill, he had not felt fully awake until he, or someone else, had shaved him. He was a fastidious man by nature who took pride in his still muscular, youthful body. He always liked to look his best when confronting the day. Confronting was absolutely the correct word. Savoring the challenges of each new day, he had looked the attractive, fit opponent. But today he could not shave. Instead, he put back the shaving cream that he had taken from the medicine chest and closed the cabinet door softly.

One last glance in the mirror, and then he must return to bed. He searched the image for his face as he had known it all these years without the effects of medication and the weariness of illness. Of his features, he recognized only his eyes. They were still icy blue and intensely alert. As he watched his reflection, he saw his face dissolve until only the eyes were visible. Edward felt startled—something was not right, and he wanted to leave but could not tear his gaze away from the enormous blue eyes of the stranger now looking at him. Where a moment ago his own blue eyes had seemed alert, open, and questioning, these new eyes seemed stormy, rejecting, and demanding. They were set in a mask the color of bleached bone, and a vivid red mouth parted into a snarl, exposing teeth filed to razor sharpness. The mouth was laughing at him. Of that, he was sure, even though there was no sound. The face was grotesque and terrifying. In panic, Edward covered the mirror with a towel. He felt completely beaten, and he hurried awkwardly to the safety of his bed. The mask did not follow him, much to Edward's relief.

For several days, Edward told no one of his frightening experience. He was too deeply ashamed, and he was more worried than he had ever been during the last six months because he realized now that the image he had seen was the creation of his own mind. Maybe he would be able to tolerate whatever physical limitations were going to become permanent as a result of the multiple sclerosis, but how on earth was he going to tolerate insanity? Hallucinations were for people on street drugs, or for people who had serious psychiatric problems, not for solid, capable people who had never even considered the possibility of being mentally ill.

The hallucination did not return, but Edward continued to worry about it and was afraid to uncover the mirror. When he did not volunteer any information about the covered mirror, his nurse asked him what that was all about. She had noticed he was not taking care of his appearance as usual. Was he growing a beard? And even if he were, there certainly was no need to cover up the mirror in the bathroom. Edward blurted out the whole story, expecting the nurse to recoil from him. Instead, she asked him if he had reported this to the doctor.

"Of course not," was Edward's reply. "I don't want him thinking of me as a crackpot."

"But you are withholding medical information that may be important," his nurse soothed. "Hallucinations like this sometimes occur as a result of medication, and the doctor needs to know that, so I am going to call him and tell him, if you won't do it."

The relief Edward felt was beyond anything he had ever experienced. It simply had not occurred to him that bizarre experiences like this one could be medication related. Somehow he had assumed all the side effects would be physical ones, like being too restless to sleep. The doctor left instructions for Edward to continue decreasing his medication as planned and to call him if he noticed any peculiar changes in the way he was feeling.

Edward's spirits lifted as he found he was sleeping better and beginning to take off some of the extra weight he had accumulated during the last six months. Then, like a roller coaster, his spirits plummeted as he felt himself getting weaker and less energetic. Life just could not go on like this, and he had absolutely no way of knowing how to change any of it. He lost interest in almost everything, and became abrupt with the people trying to help him. The harder they tried to help, the harder Edward pushed them away. One day, his nurse told him she was resigning from her post and she would stay on only until he had found a replacement. When he asked why, she told him that he simply was so ill-humored and abusive she could see no reason to stay. Edward was crushed; he faced the sober reality that he could not be assured of the help he needed even if he paid for it. His doctor also seemed to lose interest in his welfare and could not be reached as easily on the phone anymore. In place of personal discussions on the phone with the doctor, he found he was now having them with the receptionist—and she could not really help. His children told him that he was looking much better, and that they needed to return to their own lives. Only one of them had bothered with him anyway, Edward thought angrily, so by all means they should go back to their own concerns.

That night, Edward decided that life had become a meaningless, humiliating struggle to get from the beginning of the day to the end of it. He was so pained and frustrated by his limitations that he had trouble even remembering what it was like to get up at the beginning of a day feeling well, to work for ten hours, and still have energy to socialize and enjoy himself after he left his office. His friends were remarkably loyal, and they stayed in touch with him by telephone and letter, but he missed having daily contact with a score of interesting, productive men and women. He was not feeling like much of a man at all. No work life, no social life, no will or energy to resist the tedium of failing health.

At this moment, he felt hopeless. And so intensely did he envy those who were well, it made him weep. Usually he was not given to self-pity. He would ask himself what he could do for himself, not why did this have to happen to me. Tonight he was not asking anything, feeling consumed by rage, and bereft of solace. It was possible to feel hatred for all the people who threw away their health on alcohol, overeating, and lack of exercise, who lived lives that were not very productive. But here he was helpless, after trying hard to be a decent, useful person who employed good judgment about taking care of himself. It just did not seem fair or necessary that he should be cut off from so much of what he valued in himself.

If he were to die now, it dawned on him, he would not just be a helpless puppet anymore. Could it actually be that he was thinking of suicide—of running away from having to deal with more than he could handle? Edward had always considered people who took their own lives to be very weak and unworthy. Now here he was—feeling undeservedly wretched, and unable to manage his life with the grace and style he usually mustered—for the first time actively considering what it would be like to kill himself. At first impression it seemed an interesting possibility, and one that made him feel rather calm. After all, he could plan and control his own demise very carefully. What was the protocol of suicide? He would want any attempt he made to be fatal. It would need to be as neat as possible, and somehow he would have to arrange it so that strangers, or the authorities would find him. He would not want to suffer while dying, he was suffering while living, and the point to suicide would be to end his suffering.

After he made his mental lists of do's and don'ts, he began sorting through various methods. Being an ingenious and methodical researcher, it was short work to come upon two methods that he felt would meet all the criteria, except the last; as far as he was aware, using the means which were available to him there was no way to die without suffering. He felt very pleased with himself for approaching his task so systematically, and for arriving at two possible resolutions to his predicament. Neither was elegant, but both seemed to be efficient. He would have to think about it a bit more tomorrow, but he had the feeling he would sleep well tonight.

In the morning, his housekeeper arrived with an arm-load of flowers from her garden. She asked how Edward was feeling and commented that he looked rested. He chatted warmly with her for a few minutes, thinking with affection of how well she cared for him, even though she had not been blessed with an easy life herself. He regretted all the times in the last months that he had been curt with her. As she arranged the flowers in an attractive vase, she interrupted Edward's reading to remark that it was good to see him when he was not feeling cranky. Her understatement of the anger underlying his moods amused Edward.

Today he was not feeling at all "cranky." Just the reverse, in fact. For the first time in months, he felt expansive. The day looked warm, just right for tennis—too bad he would not be able to enjoy it on the courts. He called a friend whom he had not seen in quite awhile to inquire if he were free for lunch. The date was quickly made, and he instructed his housekeeper to prepare lunch for two. After lunch, he thought, would be early enough to review the plans of the previous evening.

Edward felt almost content during most of the day. When evening arrived, he thought long and hard about the improvement in his mood, wondering how it had come about, and if it would remain. Funny how acting in a characteristically efficient manner helped him want to live. The real terror of his experiences of fury and defeat was that they were not in his customary repertory. Even so, when these feelings had the upper hand, there was no mistaking or denying them. By nature, Edward thought of himself as a patient man, but he had been suffering for long months now. He could not keep the rage from boiling over any longer. It was really too important to him. The rage was his protest to anyone who would listen, against the rotten hand fate had dealt him.

Edward found that his good mood of the day was vanishing under the weight of the seething, powerful anger that was on the verge of exploding. Maybe that was what had happened last night as he laid suicide plans. No . . . well, at least, he was not sure, but he thought his suicidal thoughts and plans were comforting because he could use his researcher's knack for anticipating problems and dispelling them, and in so doing rediscover part of himself. He could take control in a familiar way and thus have a shield against a life that was now unpredictable and frightening. He wondered if anyone really understood how much emotional pain he was in, and how much effort it took to simply go on in a life where everything had become a struggle. It was sad to think that the only time in six months he felt like himself—like he was living today—was when he was planning to give up the struggle to invest in tomorrow. Never before in his life had he been so close to quitting. Closing his eyes in hopes of merciful sleep that night, Edward wondered if he and his body could cooperate one more day in the fight for meaning. He was tired, afraid, and alone, but if he could hold onto the idea of himself as he used to be, he might make it another day.

COMMENTARY

Anger, in many forms, is a natural part of the emotional response to chronic illness. It is dormant at certain stages, surfaces at other stages, and is likely to be most prominent at predictable junctures. Anger will not be evident during the crisis stage, when the entire organism is concentrated on survival; it is, in a sense, an emotional luxury that can only exist after survival is no longer in question. Even when energy is available for anger, it still may not appear in dramatic form if the patient is frightened of losing support by expressing it (as was Evie, in her isolation), or if the person is so frightened of anger that he can't even acknowledge its existence.

Patients are most vulnerable to anger during any period of worsening of their illness—such as Edward is experiencing. Rage may be the only emotion powerful enough to counterbalance the fear that comes with worsening. Add to this, frustration with caretakers and medical impotence and the anger may be powerful indeed. Each time illness assaults the patient's self-confidence and forces him to relinquish a bit more of the dream that his illness will go away, the emotional storm of this stage is repeated. If the patient can begin to expect of himself only what is within his power to do, rather than berate himself for not being able to turn back the hands of the clock, he will be less tormented each time the anger phase is encountered.

Anger can be healthy or unhealthy, constructive or destructive.* It can be energy producing; it can be used to focus one's efforts, to control what is controllable, to walk when walking is very difficult, to undergo a demanding physical regimen. It is unhealthy only when the patient's self-esteem has been so diminished during the course of illness that he turns the anger inward, and therefore defeats himself through self-contempt, self-disgust, self-blame, and hopelessness. It is primarily this form of destructive rage that Edward is experiencing.

Remember that Edward's first impulse upon standing up is to scream. We can well imagine it to be the scream of

---

*There is a category of patients characterized by the consistent hostile use of anger as a weapon against others. These emotionally abusive patients have to be viewed differently. In nearly all cases, they have always had abusive personalities, and their anger cannot be properly viewed as a result of illness. The best approach with these patients is to be very firm and consistent with limits, and to deny them the chance to have access to caretakers with whom they are being abusive. This approach is no different from the way a caring parent would regard a child having a tantrum.

complete outrage that most of us used to good advantage as youngsters when, according to our view of the world, we had been wronged. It is precisely this type of defiant condemnation of fate that gripped Edward when he could not walk smoothly and found himself precariously balanced. In the desire to scream there is also great fear—the fear that we have all experienced as children, if not later on in adulthood—the fear of not being able to take care of oneself. In itself, the scream is perfectly understandable—a release of rage, a letting off of steam that does no damage to Edward or to anyone else. The problem is that Edward's self-esteem is very fragile. Between the damage caused by illness and by a personality that is rather rigid, he continued turning the rage inward.

Objectively, Edward's expression of rage is out of proportion to his life circumstances. He has friends, family, money, and a variety of caretakers to look after him. But Edward uses none of these resources as a means of improving his assessment of himself. His rigidity, his tendency to see things as black or white, makes him very vulnerable to attacks on his self-esteem, not only from his illness, but from his own judgments of himself. He has not allowed any of his resources—personal or monetary—to help him express his anger in overt, non-self-destructive ways. He cried to no one, he bickered a little with his nurse but without addressing his anguish, and, in general, treated the people around him as if they were invisible. This is very poor management of the torment he is feeling. He has lost all sense of perspective. Edward has a number of immediate social contacts, yet he is aware only of himself—indeed he sees only a fragment of himself—namely, the fragment he judges worthless. And he lets this fragment take over his entire life. He hangs on very tightly to the idea that he is worthless. If Edward had a more flexible personality, he would be able to tolerate a more complex view of himself than the simple judgment that he has no value. Life indeed has changed, and Edward must learn to be more realistic about what he should expect of himself. Otherwise, his self-esteem will continue to crumble. Illness is a devastatingly depriving experience, but we see in Edward what happens when the patient tries to be more powerful than the illness by being more destructive than it is.

Edward could have used some of his many resources to channel the understandable rage he is feeling into an energizing force. He could have called on his colleagues to help him stay abreast of what was going on at work; he could have energetically called on family for diversion and relief from his obsession with illness; he could have asked his doctor for the name of a counselor or therapist to whom he could have expressed his anguish, or for the names of other patients who sometimes make themselves available as telephone buddies to others in similar physical distress; he could have contacted his local MS society to find out what they could offer him. Any of these contacts would have brought Edward some enrichment to his life. Instead, his concealment of his fear, and his reluctance to admit to his emotional distress, grew out of coping mechanisms that were no longer applicable. This was not an easily structured problem in the lab. It was a problem in his life.

Edward in his pre-illness days was extremely orderly; he liked everything to be shipshape, and had very high standards for himself in his work life. These traits were quite useful in his profession, but adaptation to illness requires more of a person. It particularly requires flexibility and patience in the face of the unpredictable. The unknown is the primary fear of mankind. Edward is particularly vulnerable to this fear because all his life he has tried so hard to mask it. Unpredictability and disorder had no place in his personal universe before the illness. Edward always wanted to be in control. Following his illness he felt the control he had worked so hard to achieve was shattered. Control mistakenly meant to Edward only the manipulation of his environment, rather than the flexible emotional response to uncertainty.

Another complicating factor in Edward's situation is the particular medication he was taking. Sometimes drugs that are medically required have the unfortunate side effect of producing a feeling of being psychologically out of control. Ignorance about the side effects may make the feeling of loss of control doubly upsetting to patients and family. Edward's hallucination is a case in point. Lacking the information that hallucinations are sometimes medication related, Edward's logical mind could assume only one possibility— that he was going crazy. To Edward, the scientist, any hint that his emotions were capable of altering his perceptions of the physical world was highly alarming. And, in fact, Edward's resolve to go on with the daily struggle against the illness was shaken.

Although the hallucination was triggered by the steroids he was taking, the form it took gives us clues about Edward's innermost feelings. In place of his own reflection Edward thought he saw a blue-eyed ghoul with pointed teeth. These features were set in a face of stark, masklike whiteness, and the ghoul seemed to be both laughing at him and threatening him. One way to interpret this image is that it represents Edward's selection of himself as the primary target of his anger at being ill and the attendant loss of control. The ghoul is frightening and intends Edward harm, as does his multiple sclerosis. Its blue eyes were like his own in some ways, but were quite different in their malevolent gaze. Edward regarded himself malevolently: he judged himself helpless, pitiful, and unmanly. Thus the portion of Edward that regarded the ravages of illness with disgust, rather than sympathy, was reflected in the eyes of the ghoul. The jagged row of teeth seems a straightforward threat of harm to come. The masklike whiteness of the face is a bit more complicated. It may suggest the pallor of death. It is also likely that the whiteness is a symbol for the medical world that has so gravely disappointed Edward. He is not happy with medicine because it cannot help enough. In the world of hallucination, Edward's disappointment comes back to him in the guise of a medical masklike whiteness ridiculing him.

Edward's mind transformed his feelings of anger, helplessness, and fear into a hallucination that graphically displayed for him just how angry (murderously angry) he was feeling. He resorted to the magical technique of covering the mirror and not telling anyone about his experience in hopes that this could in some way control the hallucination. Covering the mirror is a dramatic illustration of how Edward seeks control through covering anger and fear rather than by flexible coping. But the damage was already done because he began to question his sanity along with his ability to be a purposeful and worthwhile individual.

From this point on, Edward experienced an escalation of misdirected anger (anger directed at himself rather than the disease) and clung more desperately than ever to his desire for unrealistic control. These responses culminated in thoughts about suicide.

The loss of an idea about how life is going to progress, coupled with the loss of control over bodily capabilities, is devastating to the chronically ill. The ability to control something—to predict anything—seems of paramount importance to patients, often replacing the more accurate assessment of how they are functioning on a daily basis. A patient who, like Edward, has done extremely well with his illness over many years, begins to think, "If I cannot make this symptom go away, life is not worth living." Patients using this logic are actively collaborating with their illness to destroy the possibilities for preserving quality in their lives.

With Edward, this collaboration is rather apparent. He is shattered by having to change his lifestyle to such a marked degree. These losses are very real, and they need to be mourned. One phase of a particular lifestyle has come to an end—and it hurts. However, it is a very big jump from the immediate pain to the thought of permanently giving up. (Temporary episodes of what looks like giving up are usually only times of mourning and regrouping.) What then triggered Edward's suicidal thoughts? As has been previously mentioned, Edward is a rigid man who needs to put things in their proper pigeonholes, and illness defies pigeonholing. He has an exaggerated need for control, a part of his pre-illness personality. But even with these traits, something more basic than the physical symptoms of illness was threatening Edward's ability to survive the trauma of illness. In some cases, the crucial issue undermining the patient's resources might be a disruption of family support, loss of spiritual or religious faith, or the financial disaster brought on by illness. In Edward's case, it seems to involve questions about his sanity during and following the terrifying hallucination he had. For Edward, his mind was his most prized attribute. To lose faith in one's sanity while attempting to adapt to the rigors of illness, has thrown many patients into despair.* When Edward experienced the hallucination—something he was completely unprepared for, and over which

---

*Questions regarding one's sanity may originally be suggested by doctors (either intentionally or unintentionally). It is very common in illness with initial symptoms that are vague, for patients to go to doctors and be dismissed as having too much stress in their lives.

he felt total lack of control, his faith in himself as a rational man was severely shaken.

The rational side of Edward thrived on planning—the scientist's life. Instead of using his skills to design a study, he used them to plot his own demise. That he turned the constructive desire for planning and control to such destructive use was a function of his anger. The inappropriateness of turning his anger against fate inward on himself was not noticed by Edward. The overwhelming intensity of his despair, a lifelong habit of seeing himself as needing to be perfect, his current belief that he might be crazy, all helped produce this misdirected control attempt.

That Edward is angry is seen throughout his story. He is angry about everything and at everyone, and he has ceased to be aware of how much he is the beneficiary of others' attentions. Family, helpers, and friends may also be thoroughly exhausted and angry as well. For everyone involved, anger is an alternative to fear. And no one with this degree of fear should be expected to deal with it by himself.

There is, however, an early constructive action that one can take to cope with this anger and fear: one can seek the aid of a mental health specialist. Patients, and those close to them, must feel free to seek emotional relief through such a specialist, and should have no reluctance in asking a physician for a referral to a therapist. Doctor, patient, and family must view referral as another tool against the ravages of illness. Contact between the doctor and patient is preserved, not threatened by referral; neither patient nor doctor is abandoning the partnership between them if a mental health specialist is consulted. The team is being expanded so that the distinction between the illness and the person is underscored. The illness is what made it hard for Edward to walk. At the point where Edward judged he was nothing more than the illness, it was Edward who might have made it impossible for him to live. There are many positive choices that can be made using the same energy Edward put into almost giving up. It seems his flirtation with suicide helped him resolve to struggle on. He would do well to be using a therapist to help him discover other, less treacherous, ways to strengthen this resolve.

CHAPTER FOUR

RECONSTRUCTION

Peter Brown was acutely aware that this was only the third hour since his last medication—it would be an hour before he could expect relief from pain. The post-surgical discomfort that had awakened him had now progressed to intense pain. If he could distract himself, he could stall the leap from intense pain to severe pain. The night nurses, he knew, could not dispense extra medication without a doctor's approval. By the time he finished complaining, and the nurses finished going through channels, it would be time for his customary medication and nothing would have been gained.

It was now two o'clock in the morning of his second post-operative day. Peter was no stranger to hospitals, but he had never learned how to simply pass time while waiting to recover from surgery. Looking hopefully about the room for some distraction, he noted with supreme boredom the dull green walls, the uninviting washstand, and the curtain dividing his side of the room from that of the other occupants.

Fortunately, Peter's side had the window, and he looked through the dirty screen at cloudy skies dimly lit by street lamps from somewhere below his second-story room. During the day he could sometimes see a bird or two, but in the middle of the night he could see nothing. Peter's boredom was pierced by a clattering sound as a maintenance cart was wheeled outside the room. The two men pushing the cart talked in normal street tones, as if they were shopping downtown during the middle of the day. Loudly a nurse told them to quiet down. The clattering and clanking continued.

Peter felt outraged that the hospital's patients were never allowed to sleep in peace. The night noise of the hospital was almost as bad as the daytime noise. There were times when he wanted to read the riot act to the whole lot of them, from chief administrator to cook, for their lack of consideration. He was in pain, and they could not even provide a hospital where he could suffer in peace. "I don't know why I'm surprised," Peter said to himself. "This is my third surgery in this hospital and I've never been permitted to rest."

At 45, surgery for Crohn's disease was more worrisome than his initial surgery at 22 had been. Crohn's disease is an inflammation of the intestinal tract of unknown cause with an uncertain prognosis. Several types of treatment were available, and depending on how well the patient tolerated them, life could often go on fairly well. But in the middle of an episode, everything came to a halt. The disease was enormously painful. Digestion was not handled smoothly by the inflamed intestine, even if one's diet were rigidly controlled, and diarrhea and painful gas-induced bloating gave the patient little peace. At its worst, the disease could be incapacitating, since pain and weakness were early symptoms in acute episodes. The weakness progressed because the ailing intestine could digest fewer and fewer nutrients.

Peter's most recent attack had begun abruptly a few weeks after he learned he would not receive the promotion he thought he deserved. His boss had decided to promote a man for whom Peter had little respect, and who could, he knew, do the job no better than he. Peter had objected to the other's impending promotion, but when he became seriously ill, he knew he had lost whatever chance there might have been for his boss to reconsider his choice. Before long, Peter was on a medical leave, supporting his family with disability insurance, and facing his worst experience with Crohn's to date. Early trials on medication failed, and a change to a liquid diet supplemented with a special nutrient drink was ordered. The special formula was a powdered concoction that smelled like cement. No matter how Peter's wife attempted to mix the drink, it was unpalatable, with a persistent chalky taste. Powdered chocolate chalk mixed with every possible solvent was Peter's complete bill of fare for a month. Not only was there no improvement in the inflammation, it seemed to be getting worse at an alarming rate. Peter had dropped from 165 pounds to 130. He was so weak he could scarcely sit up.

When Peter became so sick that he could not consume an adequate supply of liquids, his doctor put him in the hospital, and Peter was unceremoniously informed that abdominal surgery would be scheduled as soon as his strength improved. He had lost so much blood due to the constant irritation of his intestinal lining that a transfusion was ordered immediately.

Following the transfusion and the intravenous introduction of fluids, Peter felt marginally better, but his rate of improvement soon halted, and then steadily declined. The immediate task, the doctor then informed Peter, was to reverse the weakness. He recommended a surgical procedure that made it possible to supply nutrients directly to one of the chest's main vessels. The surgery would take place the next day. Peter had severe doubts about this procedure. Indeed, he was afraid he might not survive it. Any intrusion into the chest area sounded risky at best. Nevertheless, the surgery went very smoothly, and Peter began to notice almost immediate improvement in his strength. Since he was now taking no food by mouth and his intestines were having a complete rest, his pain rapidly decreased. Ten days later he underwent major surgery for the removal of a three-foot segment of intestine. How many feet were left? he had wondered with alarm, and what would happen to him if further inflammation required more surgery? Surely one must run out of intestines at some point.

Surprising that a recollection of how he had come to be lying in a hospital bed with nothing to do made Peter want to smile. It seemed incredible to have been transformed from a ghostlike creature at death's door to a postsurgical patient recovering nicely in less than two weeks. Peter was aware that the reprehensible desire to laugh was nothing like his customary deportment—usually so sober. It was as if there was a rebel within him who, intoxicated with medication and relief, was thumbing his nose at death's premature attempt to nab him.

At this point, Peter succumbed to the unfortunate impulse to laugh and was brought up short by a ferocious stab of pain. As if on cue, the nurse bearing fourth-hour relief glided in.

"Feeling much better today, are we, Mr. Brown?"

"I feel lousy. I thought I'd never make it."

The nurse gave him his shot and quietly retreated, leaving Peter alone, his ill humor returned. A moment ago he had felt like chuckling, but the two minute interchange with the insipid nurse left him feeling furious. He would have to find a way to occupy himself, or turn into the worst crank anyone had ever seen. Peter surrendered to the effect of the drug and fell asleep.

In the morning, Peter felt much worse. He did not understand why, for him, the third day following surgery was so much more painful than the first or second days, but here was the same phenomenon again. Even though it lent little in the way of physical comfort, recognizing a pattern in his physical distress relieved his mind somewhat. Peter could hear the breakfast cart rumbling along from door to door. He managed a weak smile at the young girl whose job it was to dispense the proper tray to each patient.

"What's this morning's poison?" he quipped.

The girl didn't exactly scowl at him, but neither did she smile or return his joke. Peter sighed. The day promised to be a long one. Clearly, in this hospital, there were rules: never allow the patient to sleep peacefully, and never allow him to make light of his predicament. God, what a place. At least this slender waif had not patronized him. He would take honest irritation any day over the terrible "Now, now" that the nurses seemed to use continually to chide him for being obstreperous. Just as he had feared, breakfast was positively disgusting. He had a bite of jello—which in the hospital has a consistency of rubber cement—and left the broth untasted.

From a brief morning nap, Peter awoke to a clear wintry day, the kind he especially liked. The sun was still quite weak, but it was bright enough to make the sky appear clean and crisp. Suddenly, Peter felt like trying to walk. With the aid of nurses, he had been able to stand briefly since the night of his surgery. These initial attempts were accompanied by his howls of protest; it seemed to him unkind to inflict extra pain on a surgical patient. Despite the explanations about resuming normal sitting and standing patterns to promote healing, Peter remained unconvinced. Today, however, he wanted to get out of the railed bed and walk about.

A pleasant voice over the intercom speaker answered his call.

"Yes, Mr. Brown?"

"Is there anyone currently on escort duty? I feel like a walk."

"We will be happy to oblige after lunch."

"I will look for you about 12:30 then," Peter replied.

Peter now had one hour and 45 minutes to kill. His neighbor was watching one of those abominable soap operas where all the surgical patients look as if they have just stepped out of a limousine on their way to a presidential reception. Never a tube in sight. Such rot. A paper had been delivered to his room, and he scanned the headlines. Seeing an item of interest, he read on. A friend of his was heading up a volunteer jazz band to play for town functions or for service agencies such as convalescent hospitals or schools for handicapped children. Peter wondered, almost hesitantly, if they could use a rusty drum player. He had played in college and in those days was pretty good. His wife, Lorraine, had encouraged him to continue playing, but at the same time had never neglected to remind him that the apartment walls were thin, or that one of their two young children was asleep. Scheduling became such a problem that Peter eventually found no way to practice. Even so, the drums had never been sold or put away.

It seemed he had been defending those drums from childhood on. His father had hated them, so Peter, in rebellion, became a diligent student who practiced at every opportunity. It had been satisfying to defy his father in this way. But when he wanted to major in music, his father laid down the law: his college education would be funded only for something practical. Peter submitted and took up engineering. Physics and thermodynamics did nothing for his soul, and he later changed to computer programming, then a somewhat novel field and, to Peter, strangely akin to music. He never really understood this connection, but he felt the same ease when he picked up his drum sticks as when he attempted to write a program for some sticky problem.

On graduation, he had several job offers. Unfortunately, he had again taken his father's advice to choose the most established company because no one knew what a start-up company would do. The start-up company he had rejected was making millions, and the established firm became stodgier and less current with recent developments all the time. Peter's problem with Crohn's disease started the year after he began working for the firm that still employed him.

He still had half an hour before his walk. He opened the bedside table and withdrew some scented travel wipes and began to cleanse himself as well as he could. Feeling refreshed—more the product of optimism than of physical strength—Peter awaited his escort in white.

After a while, Peter was not so sure that he wanted to go walking. His early morning enthusiasm for fitness had waned under the strain of increasing pain and fatigue. Before he could do anything to ward off the arrival of the two nurses who would help him out of bed, the cavalry arrived, brisk in starched uniforms. Peter's spirits sagged, but he resolved to go through with his adventure.

"Ready for a stroll, Mr. Brown?" The nurse was relaxed and smiling as she expertly turned back the bedclothes.

"I think so. The question is, are the two of you really ready to help me complete the marathon course?" Peter's comment was partially serious. He was a tall man compared to the 5'2" women who were to be his supports.

"Just swing your legs to the floor, but don't put any weight on them yet." Peter did as he was told, even though the movement caused sharp pain.

"Shift your weight gradually onto your feet and stand up when you are ready, Mr. Brown."

Peter liked the nurse who was doing all the talking. She gave him the feeling that she knew exactly what was going to happen and that he would survive it, despite his doubts. The nurse did not flinch when Peter let out an involuntary bellow of pain as his body rebelled against having to use muscles temporarily injured by surgery.

"Now try a step or two. Just small ones and we will walk around the bed."

Peter, surprised that each shuffling step seemed less difficult than the last, began smiling like a young boy who had just been told he would be getting his favorite ice cream for dessert. After reaching the foot of the bed, Peter wanted to go into the halls where he knew there were railings on the walls and he could walk without help.

"We'll go into the hall, but we'll stay with you today," the nurse said.

Peter would have felt angrier at this curbing of his enthusiasm if he hadn't suddenly begun to tire dramatically. With a sense of considerable relief, Peter was eased back into bed only to become aware of extreme fatigue from his exertions, and an increase in the stubborn pain inside him. He asked the nurse for a pain killer. As he took his pill, she busied herself with a triangular metal bar hanging from a track running above his bed.

"As you can see, Mr. Brown, you may slide this to wherever it will do you the most good. If you feel like exercising, you have an impromptu gymnasium at your disposal. You can do a lot for yourself without even getting out of bed."

Peter was quick to understand what the nurse meant. "Modified leg ups?" When she smiled at him, Peter nodded appreciatively.

Later that afternoon, Peter found that if he moved very cautiously, he could slip a leg through the triangle so that the bar supported the back of his knee. Then he could, with considerable effort and not inconsiderable pain, move his leg up and down. Mindful of his still fragile abdominal muscles, Peter was careful not to overtax himself, and he was nearly through with what he thought to be an appropriate exercise period when his wife came through the door.

Lorraine was a calm, competent woman whose only real flaw, Peter thought, was a slightly sour disposition. Lorraine had been a pillar of support during the months of severe illness, very capably handling the family's finances, her own job, and visits to Peter. She and Peter had matter-of-factly discussed how to curb expenses during the time Peter was on medical leave and how best to handle his convalescence so that it would not be too hard on Lorraine or the family. They had agreed Peter should stay in the hospital as long as his doctor was willing so that the expenses would be almost completely covered by his company's insurance plan. Lorraine had been sensible and supportive throughout all these discussions, gently but firmly guiding Peter away from his fanciful notions that he would be back on his feet and working within a week. Understandable wishful thinking, Lorraine had soothed, but he really should give himself enough time to recover before going back to the stress of a job he no longer enjoyed. It was simply too much for Lorraine when she walked into the room and spotted Peter exercising away, albeit in slow motion, as if nothing in the world were amiss.

"Peter! For heaven's sake, stop that right away!" Lorraine shrilled.

Peter, who was about to cease his exertions anyway, immediately desisted. "It's not the end of the world, Lorraine—"

He was going to go on and explain himself, but instead he began to laugh—a true belly laugh. Peter alternately hooted with merriment and groaned with pain.

"I guess you shouldn't make me laugh yet. But you looked so funny, I couldn't help it."

Lorraine was befuddled; she didn't know if she should be alarmed, so she just stood there, irresolute. Then she began to giggle—Peter's laugh was really infectious.

The burst of laughter eventually melted away, and Peter tried to greet his wife in a more customary fashion. Lorraine was not ready to be completely assuaged, and a bit of her self-righteous indignation returned when she asked for an explanation of the amazing event she had witnessed upon entering the room.

"It's really very simple," replied Peter. "I am getting bored and restless. When I was walking with the nurses today, I could see how weak I've become and one of the nurses showed me the triangle and suggested it might be helpful."

"Will you please ask the doctor if it's all right?"

Peter nodded. "I was going to do that anyway, and I also want to know if there's anything special he can think of to help me get back on my feet. I really don't want to go through this again, and I have the feeling it will take more than exercise to keep me from landing back here again in a few years."

The meeting with the doctor was at six that evening. Peter's gastroenterologist was an energetic, authoritative man whose 30 years of experience gave credibility to his remarks. He was self-assured, congenial, and matter-of-fact. Peter had always liked Dr. Elker, and genuinely believed that he had always listened carefully to what the doctor told him. He was especially interested in his doctor's current appraisal of the medical problems and how Peter could minimize them. Dr. Elker entered the room with an unhurried, but purposeful stride. He examined his patient and asked him how he was feeling. Dr. Elker pulled up a chair and told Peter he was recovering nicely.

"Anything on your mind, Peter?"

"Quite a bit, actually. I really want to get out of here, and I don't want to find myself here again for further surgery. There must be something more that I can do to protect myself."

Dr. Elker patiently reviewed for Peter advice that he had been giving him for 23 years. Peter must look to improving the overall quality of his life. There was no one thing that was medically indicated to stamp out vulnerability to Crohn's disease; the mechanism of the disease appeared to be quite complicated. But as long as Dr. Elker had known Peter, there had been major sources of tension in Peter's life that should be eliminated.

Dr. Elker's comments were not new to Peter, but this time he listened with a very different attitude. In the past, Peter had felt he was merely a victim of circumstance, unable to do anything but what he was doing. How does one reduce stress in a world characterized by stress? The prescription to relax sounded fine, but Peter had never found a way to do it. Tonight, however, he was a far more receptive listener than usual. The doctor's words did not simply go in one ear and out the other. Peter asked him to point out the areas of stress he had observed, and he had to agree with the doctor that there were problems on the job, unnecessary tensions between him and Lorraine, often when there was no realistic crisis, and—harder to face—problems in himself concerning what he wanted to do and how uncomfortable he felt when he needed to speak out.

Peter also asked about exercise. He was told that as long as nothing hurt sharply he could work out a program of gradually increasing exercise for himself. The sooner he started, and the more dedicated he was, the better the progress would be. When Peter asked about diet, Dr. Elker surprised him by telling him that he could gradually vary the bland diet he had been observing for years to see how he would tolerate other food items. The main thing was to eat a series of small meals during the day. Vitamin supplements were recommended, as was the avoidance of caffeine, alcohol, and smoking. As he had done before, Dr. Elker reminded Peter that this advice was what most doctors were now giving to encourage patients to make a significant investment in future good health. What the direct effect on the Crohn's disease would be, Dr. Elker could not say, but he could say with certainty that if these guidelines were observed, and if moderation was the basic rule of thumb, Peter's overall health would be improved. The unmistakable emphasis in all the doctor's remarks was on the quality of life, both now and in the future.

Quality of life was also the primary concern for Peter now. A part of him that usually remained silent had chorused a series of yeses to Dr. Elker's outline of changes needed in Peter's work life, his family life, and in his own feelings about himself. A combination of fear and exhilaration gave Peter yet another bad night. Dr. Elker had pointed the way to altering his life, but knowing himself to be a person who avoided change, Peter felt fearful. On the other hand, the doctor's comments had given Peter a vibrant sense of power because he realized that he had choices. The idea was almost stunning. "I am not a mere victim," Peter told himself, "and I can choreograph the changes I wish to make."

The last days in the hospital were ones of smooth recovery from surgery and a gradual increase in his sense of physical strength. Peter spent some of his remaining time in the hospital making notes on long-and short-range plans for effecting changes in his life. The activity made the time pass quickly and helped him think clearly. It made him feel good to plan his life—efficient, productive, doing something for himself. It was a beginning!

At one level, Peter was occasionally aware that all his plans and efforts might not make any difference in the progression of his illness. But he thought he was beginning to see some merit in a favorite motto of his children: Live in the here and now. The boys, when home from college, had tried in vain to explain what this saying meant, but Peter had felt it was a way of avoiding responsibility and commitments. This philosophy seemed to fly in the face of Peter's lifelong practice of self-denial, and of choosing the safe rather than the fulfilling route. But perhaps his children were only suggesting that if he lived each day fully, he would be happier and less frustrated. Even with his new-found enthusiasm, Peter suspected that to strike a balance between living fully in the present, and flexible planning for the future, would be an ongoing struggle. Old habits, he realized, did not change easily, but as Dr. Elker had suggested, change became easier when the rewards of new behavior became evident.

After his discharge from the hospital, Peter sorted through his notes on how to change his life. The ones he had spent the most time on concerned possible ways to alter his work situation. This would take serious long-range planning and couldn't be done swiftly, but he could begin to act in another area—recreation, for instance. Many of the activities that interested him were not suitable to a convalescent. Jogging, for example, was going to have to wait. He really wanted something he could do now. The slip marked music had the name and phone number of his friend Lou Rose on it. Lou was an architect who played the saxophone and was heading up the volunteer civic band. Peter dialed the number quickly, before he lost his nerve.

"Hello, Lou? Peter Brown here."

"Peter! Good to hear from you, how are things?"

"I think I am doing pretty well, thanks. I'm calling about one of your projects."

"Which one?" laughed Lou, who was always in the midst of several projects at once.

"Well, I saw the announcement about the band. What kind of response have you had?"

"For a good idea, the response has been kind of slow, but we have a group of people who are interested in beginning to rehearse. We could still use more horns."

"How about a back-up drummer?" Peter asked.

"I was hoping you would ask, but why back-up?"

"I don't know. It's been a long time since I played, and there are times, as you know, when my health gives out and I can't do much of anything."

"That's not much different from anyone else," Lou said. "We have a young dentist who covers emergencies for everyone else in town. He might have to leave in the middle of a performance. Everyone else is as out of practice as you are— the main point is just to have fun. We're going to meet in two weeks, by the way. Why not come over and meet everyone?"

Peter promised to drop by, if he were feeling up to it. The next step was to tell Lorraine. He knew by the amount of dread he felt that he expected her to react negatively, and he was afraid he wouldn't be able to defend his position. It was just something he wanted to try. For a generous, kindhearted woman, how was it that Lorraine always made him feel so inadequate and guilty? He realized that he was not being accurate or fair. She made him feel guilty only when he attempted to do anything new. She did not make him feel guilty about his bouts with illness or, for that matter, his bouts of depression and bad humor. He never got truly angry, but when he was sick, he had to admit he was very irritable. Lorraine withstood his lack of appreciation of her efforts, his endless complaining about his job. She never made the mistake of trying to cheer him up by robbing him of his complaints, but was always there as a levelheaded and sympathetic listener. When he became overly self-indulgent she told him so without malice.

He and Lorraine were good partners in the sense that they worked well together raising the children, taking care of their home, and making family plans. Each respected the wishes and feelings of the other, and, even if their marriage had lost some of its earlier zip and joy, both spouses were content in the knowledge that they loved each other.

Why, then, was he so sure that Lorraine would be disapproving of his plans to resume playing the drums, and why did he feel afraid to rock the boat? Anything new rocked the boat, but Peter couldn't tell if he were in a rowboat or a steamer. He and Lorraine had always been careful not to create surprises in their lives. At times, Peter was very aware that Lorraine's reliance on habit was one of the characteristics that had attracted him to her. She had reminded him of the way things were handled in his family, and that had felt very comfortable. She did not mock him for succumbing to his father's demand that he change majors in college, but had applauded him for doing the sensible, if not the actually necessary, thing. The more Peter reflected on his highly satisfactory marriage, the more he had thought it likely that he and Lorraine were good mates because they both feared novelty. Now he was thinking of making a host of major changes in his life, and he did not want to lose Lorraine in the process. He comforted himself with the idea that he had two weeks before the meeting and could pick the right moment to talk to her.

Then his gaze traveled to the drums in the corner. If he didn't speak now, he would simply continue looking at the drums rather than playing them. He felt relieved when he resolved to bring the subject up at lunch.

Lorraine was a capable cook who had tackled the project of introducing real food gradually into Peter's diet with enthusiasm. Since he still could not handle foods that were very high in roughage, or that contained seeds or nuts, she designed meals that were plainer than their usual fare, but which were attractive and nourishing. She regretted the loss of asparagus, bran muffins, and raspberry jam, but if Peter minded, he did not complain.

Lunch consisted of a tasty omelet. While buttering his toast, Peter told Lorraine he had some news to share.

"What's up?" she inquired, searching his face for clues.

"I think I've come up with a way to follow Dr. Elker's advice to relax more." Peter was a little shamefaced; he knew this was a statement designed to lessen his anxiety, and set Lorraine up as Dr. Elker's adversary if she disapproved of his idea.

"You don't seem very relaxed just now." Lorraine commented. Lorraine was not combative, but she was very observant, and Peter silently blessed her for opening up the topic he had been afraid to broach.

"I'm afraid you will not like the idea, and it is important to me. "

"I guess we won't know if I disapprove or not if you won't tell me what's on your mind."

Peter quickly told her how he had seen the announcement in the paper, that Lou still needed a drummer, and how it was just a fun event and not a life-or-death commitment.

Lorraine was pensive for a moment, then asked when he was going to start. When Peter told her, she abruptly flared into indignation.

"That means you are going to do exactly the same thing you've done the last two times. You are not going to give yourself time to rest and really heal from the surgery. I don't like that at all. It takes a lot of strength to play the drums. Where's your good sense gone?"

Peter let Lorraine finish. He had accidentally misled her, he said. He was not going to actually begin playing in two weeks, but was going to meet the rest of the band, if he felt up to it.

This explanation seemed to satisfy Lorraine. When she smiled, Peter knew she was not going to debate the issue with him, but had come up with a conclusion of her own.

"What's the smile about?" he asked.

"It will be good to hear the drums again, because I think if you play them you will stop tapping pencils and pens on the desk all the time. It drives me nuts."

"I didn't know that."

"And I didn't know that my disapproval causes you so much concern." Then, becoming very serious, Lorraine said, "I think we've gotten too careful with each other. Everything is so rehearsed and polite that I sometimes think we know each other less and less. You've changed since you were in the hospital this last time, and I'd like to know what kinds of changes I'll have to deal with."

"You've put your finger on what I see as the problem. You get very edgy if I suggest any kind of change."

"We become very edgy if changes are contemplated, no matter who introduces them," Lorraine retorted.

Peter was cautious. "Do you think you can stand one more change today? I've been doing a lot of thinking about a change that needs to be made in the future. It will take a lot of planning, and I don't have the solution yet."

"Sounds serious, Peter. What are you thinking?"

"I'm not sure, given the practicalities—my age and my health—how it can be done, but I want to quit my job."

"That is a big one, but if you can figure it out, it won't be a minute too soon for me. I'm sick of hearing you complain because you are so frustrated all the time. I really think you will feel better. At least you won't be furious all the time. If you can find something you like and that we can afford, I don't see how you can lose, even if the Crohn's condition does not disappear for good. For now, though, you have enough to do regaining your strength. Don't you think you are overdoing the walks up and down the driveway?"

Peter began tapping his spoon on the table and wished he felt well enough to pound the drums. "Why won't you let me make that decision? I am not a fool, and I intend to nap later today. That sort of remark isn't helpful. I know you're concerned, but why not ask me how I feel after my walk and let me tell you how I am making out."

Lorraine was somewhat startled and hurt by Peter's uncharacteristic sharpness. "I will try to make a few changes of my own, but I think you can point them out less angrily than you did just now."

"I'm not at all sure of that. Just think of all the yelling we've never done. Maybe some of it needs to come out now, for both our sakes. We don't have to agree about everything."

"We don't have to disagree about everything. Didn't Dr. Elker suggest moderation?" They smiled at each other.

COMMENTARY

When survival is no longer at stake, when the patient is no longer overwhelmed by critical symptoms of fear or anger, there may be energy available for emotional reconstruction to begin. Often a remission of symptoms, or an improvement in physical condition, precedes this stage, but not necessarily. What is necessary is a kind of equilibrium in the patient's feelings about his illness. I see patients, for example, whose disease process shows no sign of abatement who make the step from anger to reconstruction by having mastered their fear to the extent that they are no more frightened today than they were last week. Energy used to combat fear can now be directed in other ways.

During the reconstruction phase, the patient regains the feeling that he is a worthwhile individual, not just a collection of symptoms. Instead of passive victim, he feels capable of making fulfilling choices for himself, of striving for more quality in his life. I refer to reconstruction as a phase, but it is really an ongoing process in which the patient slowly, and with inevitable setbacks, rebuilds a healthy emotional life, despite physical illness.

When we meet Peter, successfully recovering from surgery, reconstruction is possible for him. He has had a lot of previous experience with his illness over the last 20 years, and there have been other reconstructions—physical recoveries after severe episodes of illness. But this time he attempts a different kind of reconstruction. In addition to physical recovery, Peter strives for emotional well-being, to enhance the quality of his life by reexamining his habitual passive stance toward life.

What signs does Peter show of emotional reconstruction? The first sign we see is irritation and indignation with hospital routine. Irritation in a patient is rarely seen as a positive emotion by caretakers, but this is a mistake. Irritability, indignation, and feisty cantankerousness can all be signs of health. Although hospital caregivers are used to labeling this behavior as negative and disruptive of routine, informally many staff people comment that it is the patients who argue and fight who do well. Furthermore Peter's anger is appropriately expressed—he doesn't fly into a rage or abuse anyone—and it has appropriate targets: the noisy orderlies, a patronizing nurse, the unnecessarily unpalatable food. Contrast Peter's anger with the self-destructive anger of Edward, which leads to depression and his flirtation with suicide. Edward directs his anger at himself, saying, I am worthless. Peter directs his anger at inadequate and insensitive treatment. His is a righteous indignation signaling an emerging sense of self-worth that says, I should not be treated this way, I deserve more. Both Peter and Edward have spent many years being angry with fate. They both have a right to feel angry; they both have lost their health. Peter, however, begins to see that he feels trapped by circumstances in his life unrelated to illness. These he has a chance of changing because what needs to change are his attitudes about himself. In life, we do have the power to control our attitudes, even when we can affect no change in circumstances.

Peter's humor is another sign of growing emotional health. Bantering with the staff, he is trying to alleviate the boredom he feels and make some social contact. Again his humor is appropriate, essentially nonhostile. The food is awful, and to joke about it is to put the situation in its proper perspective. An ability to promote, pursue, and enjoy merriment is a continual source of healing. Illness is a grim reality, but there are situations created by the illness that are inherently funny. A sense of the absurd and the comic is a major safeguard against lasting depression. Peter breaks up when he sees the comic look of surprise on Lorraine's face as she enters the room and sees him exercising. His laughter causes her to laugh, thus lightening the situation and defusing a possible argument. Here humor has created a perspective that allows husband and wife to communicate more effectively.

Another convincing sign of reconstruction is a willing and active participation in physical rehabilitation, such as Peter began in the hospital. He does not wait for others to do for him what he needs to accomplish alone. Peter is fortunate because there are specific things he can do to build up his strength. This is not always the case. Most often, though, the things a patient can do seem small and inconsequential to him. This is an error; he may not be able to make a recovery, but the small things he can do on a daily basis to preserve what is possible to preserve are quite important. The very angry or depressed patient will not be able to see this. The patient who is feeling more emotionally intact will simply see to it that he preserves and enhances what he can.

Another indication of emotional growth is Peter's changed relationship with his doctor. After 20 years, Peter is finally showing signs of being in a mature doctor-patient partnership. He is not behaving as if his doctor were a father who provides dire directives with which he, Peter, must resentfully comply. Peter is looking for new beginnings, and we see a dramatic change in how he listens to what he is told. He does not listen passively, we notice; he asks questions to get the information he needs, replacing compliance with comprehension. Peter is beginning to realize that as the patient, he must be the ultimate coordinator of all the medical attention he receives.

The doctor's final prescription for Peter is a change in lifestyle that will allow him a more manageable and fulfilling existence. Though he has heard this many times before, Peter now takes this advice seriously instead of dismissing it out of hand. He begins to see that he is not only responsible for his health, but for the quality of his life. That he believes that the goal of a more fulfilling life is attainable, and that the tasks involved do not seem overwhelming is a very hopeful sign. Peter now has the emotional resources and energy to work toward that goal. Leaving the hospital, Peter takes his first tentative steps toward that goal in his active renewal of interest in music, his future planning about more satisfying employment, and his attempts at a more attentive honest relationship with his wife.

Reconstruction is a phase characterized by hope and goal-oriented striving. For the patient to make successful strides, both patient and family must have patience, and the ability to change attitudes. How can family help? An important step is to reexamine certain attitudes. Have we, as helpers, become locked into viewing the patient a certain way? How much of the patient's conversation is tuned out because we assume he doesn't know what's best for him? Do we have less respect for his judgment and independence since his illness? It is often very hard for spouses to be supportive and nurturing partners rather than anxious, authoritarian guardians—especially when they bear the burden of finances, household chores, and childrearing, and when they are saddened and frightened by the spouse's illness. But they must remember that physical illness has not necessarily made the patient less able to think; it has just made him more reliant on others to compensate for physical limitations. Illness has provided the injury; they are adding insult to injury.

Peter and Lorraine illustrate some of these problems. Peter is sharp with Lorraine when she criticizes his rehabilitation attempts as "overdoing it." She must realize that at this point he knows what he can or cannot do, and that her overprotectiveness undermines in him a vital sense of assertiveness and independence. He must realize that she is tired and frightened and that in the past his judgment was not always so trustworthy. But the Browns are a loving couple with strong marriage bonds, and they are learning to communicate more honestly with each other without nastiness or disrespect. It is likely that they will weather this period well.

Goal-oriented striving requires flexibility and reasonable expectations. If one approach to a goal does not work, perhaps another will. Both the hope and the primary accomplishment comes from setting the goal and trying to reach it. Often reasonable goals cannot be reached without radical changes in attitude. For example, a person whose diet has been limited might conceivably have given up all socializing that involves food—a very depriving experience. He wants to resume such social contacts. If, to meet this goal, he eats the wrong foods at the expense of his health the person is not in the reconstruction phase, but still in anger. An appropriate means of achieving the goal of dining socially would be to learn about permissible cuisines and meet friends at a restaurant that serves these foods. Or even to meet friends at a restaurant and have some broth. The person is not sacrificing anything by going to the restaurant, and is gaining important social contact, but to see this requires a different mindset than that seen in earlier stages.

Peter's goal setting reflects a healthy reconstructive attitude. If he cannot jog, he still gets satisfaction from walking. If a career change must be left to the future, he creates satisfaction for himself by taking up his drums. Probably the biggest change in attitude that occurs during this stage is learning to be able to focus on the present. No amount of dwelling on the past will bring as much pleasure as the present and what it offers. Elaborate plans about the far future may create more anxiety than focusing on the near future. "Living in the here and now" became one of the mottos of the '60s. Being able to do so does not imply a selfish indulgence of one's desires at the expense of others. To do so fully really means being able to augment the present by your existence, and to reap the many moments of pleasure and fulfillment embedded in each day.

Unfortunately, some patients are unable to develop this here-and-now attitude. They deny themselves the pleasure, or relief, of the present by discounting it. To some patients the present has no meaning compared to the past (or to how they remember the past). To others, the present is denied in anticipation of future loss. These patients describe themselves as borrowing trouble. I think it is even more diminishing than that. Patients who truly cannot let themselves feel happy because they cannot stand the idea of losing this happiness have already lost it. Those who discount the present cannot be enhanced by the changes they have affected in themselves or in their environments. Perhaps the next time through the emotional cycle they will experience reconstruction more fully. But for these patients, especially if there has been a lifelong habit of not being able to really enjoy anything because they are continually battling anxiety, psychotherapy seems especially important.

Even for patients like Peter, who are truly beginning reconstruction, the problem is to strike a delicate balance in their expectations. With the exhilaration that comes from feeling effective, it is easy to forget that the disease process is a chronic one. The realistic expectation for most patients is that the physical limitations will continue to mount in some unpredictable fashion. Thus, it is critical for reconstruction that the patient understand that his emotional life does not have to shrink in direct proportion to physical limitation—that he still has opinions, attitudes, feelings, and a sense of who he is as well as a growing curiosity about who he can be.

CHAPTER FIVE

INTERMITTENT DEPRESSION

The combination of joy and pride made Stephen's heart **119** pound. The sun was brilliant and hot, beating down on the lines of dancers who moved in perfect time with the rhythms of the music. What a picture it made! Stephen loved these festivals where women and men from the distant hamlets joined in celebration with the townspeople, performing the time-honored folk dances of the past.

Stephen was leading a line of men in a precise, almost constrained dance. Up and down the line, hands looped into the crossweave of a belt hold, each man was separate yet closely aligned to his neighbors. And how strong they all looked! Stephen changed posture, as the dance moved into a new phase. Then he straightened, shoulders back and grinning, and began to call out the steps of the next sequence of the dance for those in the line. He had control of himself and the line. As the music's tempo increased, so did the swiftness and complexity of the steps Stephen called. All the men knew the music and the dance. Stephen felt his best friend moving in complete harmony with him. He had the sensation he was almost flying, and that his feet were not just his, but the entire line's. The men in his line were all between 20 and 50 years old. At 50, Stephen was one of the oldest, but he was also one of the strongest dancers. Because of his finesse, strength, and ability to blend with the music, Stephen was always asked to lead the dances at these festivals. He had always marveled at his sense of heightened aliveness, his keen pleasure in executing the precise steps to the ancient Serbo-Croatian dances. At times like these, with the line of dancers flowing behind him, he felt ecstatic.

Stephen admired the fine embroidery on the women's blouses and the long braids that fell in heavy single strands down their backs. Their faces were flushed. He was so glad that early summer had arrived and that the summer dancing had begun.

This dream of sun, pretty women, and splendid dancing was still with Stephen as he awoke. As long as he lay very still he could recapture the sounds of the music and the vision of himself happily leading the dances. A year ago, the dream had been reality. He was a very accomplished dancer, and had taken a trip to the ancient Balkan lands to study the local peasant dances. Many of them he already knew, and he made careful notations about the unfamiliar ones so that he could introduce the steps to his dance club. But shortly after returning from vacation and resuming his job on a construction team, Stephen had a stroke. This was his second. He had the first one when he was 45, and it had been a great mystery. The doctors were never able to unravel why a very healthy man with moderate blood pressure should have a stroke. It took him nearly a year to get back into shape, but he had done it. There were no lingering signs of the stroke. Determination and physical therapy had seen to that.

The doctors advised him not to return to the physically demanding work he had always done, but Stephen felt they were not being practical. What else could he do? He had a tenth-grade education and happened to love working on construction. He was a reliable worker and over the years had been promoted so that he was now the first hired and the last to be fired when work got slow. He was proud of his work record. The only time he had been out of work for health reasons occurred after he had the first stroke.

Stephen had been anxious to return to work, but he was far more anxious to return to his folk dance club—a nice assortment of people from all walks of life who had in common a love for translating emotion into dance. He had made good friends there, and he was much in demand at social gatherings because he was so accomplished.

Stephen had tried marriage—twice—and decided that he was not cut out for it. He substituted friends for the companionship of a wife and felt that he did very well. He was not lonely, and did not waste his time by drinking and watching television like other single men he knew. He could dance six nights a week in his community, and if he wanted to travel 50 miles, he could make that seven nights a week. There was always plenty going on that made him feel purposeful and content.

He'd been saving money for years to go to Europe to take a look at his father's homeland. When he fell victim to the first stroke it did not look like he would make it there. But he had fooled them all and enjoyed a marvelous adventure at the age of 48. For a lifetime he would have the memory of the trip. While he was there, Stephen had communicated in sign language most of the time. He was a stranger in a part of the world that was both curious about and resentful of strangers, but he had been treated well during the course of his travels by nearly everyone he encountered. And once he joined in the dancing he did not remain a stranger for very long.

The second stroke, like the first one, occurred without any warning. He knew that it was bad, but he also knew that he had recovered once. Now he was going to have to recover again. The right side of his body was primarily affected. He could not control the muscles of the right eye, and his face hung slack over his right cheekbone. He had trouble speaking clearly, and it seemed to him that it was harder to remember simple words than it used to be. His right arm and leg were nearly useless.

He had thrown himself into the necessary physical therapy with every ounce of strength he possessed, even though progress seemed minimal and very, very slow. He tried not to worry about the fact that the doctors could not tell him why the stroke reoccurred. They had been optimistic that the first one was a fluke. This second one meant that they had to watch him more closely and consider the possibility that the strokes were related events. Even though he used his energy to work at physical therapy, Stephen felt much more demoralized than he had been with the first stroke. He felt more vulnerable and unsure of how to protect himself. He wanted life back the way it had been—with lots of good dancing and lighthearted laughter.

The second time, like the first, the doctors marveled at Stephen's progress. He was doing much better than they had expected based on the damage from the stroke. The doctors were delighted and, for a time, so was Stephen. His progress was steady, even if it was slow. Gradually he worked the stiffness out of his hand so that he could write more legibly and eat more easily. Though he made it look easy to his observers, handling a fork was still a very difficult task, and Stephen was painfully aware of his loss of coordination and strength.

Walking was not possible at first, so there had been a wheelchair. Ever so slowly, he and the physical therapist strengthened his bad leg. Finally, there was a conversion from wheelchair to walker, and Stephen felt triumphant. At first, using the walker had been more difficult for him than climbing the scaffolding of any of the buildings he had worked on. With each step, Stephen had to consciously think about bending his knees, swinging his foot forward, and letting his weight roll from heel to toe. He could not walk and listen to someone talking to him at the same time. The rage triggered by having to think about walking, when the movements to so many complex dances were recorded somewhere in his brain and muscles, made Stephen feel so helpless and frustrated that he often wept.

Nevertheless, Stephen exercised, cursed, and sweated his way through nine months of physical therapy before he could trade in the walker for a cane. He still had to think carefully about his locomotion, and he had one foot that dragged very slightly, tending to cause him to trip. Ever watchful, Stephen relearned how to move with grace. He was pleased when his doctors or the physical therapist complimented him, and he at last felt well enough to reenter the folk dance arena.

True, he could not dance yet, but he could still participate as the person who chose the dances to be performed. He bantered with his friends between dances, changed the records, and structured everyone else's evening. It was wonderful to be back in a familiar setting with good friends drawn together by a mutual interest. Stephen always felt exhilarated while the dancing went on. His feet twitched to the rhythms, and he silently enjoyed criticizing the other dancers. The exhilaration lasted until he got home. Then, reflecting on the evening, he always arrived at the same conclusion. He hated sitting there, unable to participate, and he hated the inactivity. The loss for him was particularly cruel because he had been one of the finest dancers in the city. Even so, Stephen felt it was better to be able to socialize than to sit at home, and he could not imagine that the change would be permanent. It was unthinkable that he would never move joyfully to the call of the music.

Stephen felt that the dream he had had was much more real than his everyday life. He lay in bed for a long time recalling the dream and feeling whole. But as he awakened fully, he could not recall the simple good feelings of the dream without simultaneously feeling a sense of loss. Aside from a session with the physical therapist later that day, Stephen had no reason to get out of bed. Nearly an hour passed before he became hungry. Some days were more difficult to begin, and this one looked like it was going to be a particularly hard one. Of course, tonight was the night that there was no folk dancing, and he had a long, uneventful day stretching ahead of him.

Stephen characteristically began making a mental list of what he should do this morning. The first step was to get out of bed, then breakfast, clean up the kitchen, straighten the house. Next he had to decide whether he would go anywhere other than the physical therapist's while he was out so he could know what to wear. Shower and dress. If he made all these chores last as long as possible, he would not have to plan anything else. The morning would be gone and it would be time to leave the house. None of the items on his mental list seemed appealing, but cooking something for breakfast seemed the least appealing of all. He turned the water on to boil and poured some cereal into a bowl. As he absentmindedly began to pour the boiling water into a coffee cup, the kettle slipped through his fingers, as if he were not trying to onto hold it at all. Ever since his first stroke, Stephen had been breaking crockery when he did not have a good grasp on it, but he hadn't dropped anything in a while. And he had never dropped something as dangerous as a kettle of boiling water. Before trying to clean up the mess, Stephen's fingers sought the handle of his coffee mug. They closed around it securely. Then he lifted it and was aware of the drag on his arm from even this light weight. But he did not drop it. Somewhat mollified, he got the mop and began cleaning up the floor. The mop felt awkward and heavy in his hands. Stephen began to worry.

Replacing the mop on the service porch, he looked at the row of neatly assembled household tools on the peg board. He selected his favorite hammer—a large workman's tool with a handle worn smooth from years of use. He pulled the tray of medium-sized nails from the metal box where he kept his supplies. Armed with hammer and nails, he decided it was a very good time to mend a loose board in the fence. He was a craftsman and knew just how to use a hammer so that the tool did as much of the labor as possible. Still badly shaken by dropping the teakettle, he was intent on testing his physical powers.

The hammer felt snug and familiar in his grip. He found the place in the fence where the errant board was beginning to droop and carefully adjusted the board, placed the nail where he knew it could do the most good, and prepared to strike the head of the nail with a smart rap. In his mind's eye, he saw exactly how, with a single movement, the momentum from the swing of his arm would carry to the nail via the hammer. Smooth, precise—second nature, no problem. In reality, Stephen gripped the heavy hammer and prepared to cock his arm back for the blow, but the weight of the hammer seemed to unbalance him; it required a conscious effort to hold onto the hammer and not let it slide from his hand. His arm began to shake as muscles that were now much too weak to carry out his intention rebelled. Stephen could not believe that he was unable to will his arm to behave correctly. The evidence was certainly clear, though. It took four uncertain blows with the hammer to secure the nail. When he was finished, Stephen was exhausted, humiliated, and defeated.

Stephen went back inside feeling numb. He went to the couch to lie down, drawing a brightly colored afghan over him. He did not sleep, but lay quietly staring at the wall trying hard not to think. Some hours later, the phone rang. Stephen heard it as if from somewhere on the other side of the city. An insistent nuisance. When the phone at long last was still, the silence it created stirred Stephen. He carefully stood up and walked to the bedroom. He was so cold that the comfort of the blankets seemed very inviting. Once in bed, he again lay quietly, eyes fixed on some image from deep inside him.

Stephen missed his physical therapy appointments and folk dance gatherings for the rest of the week. If anyone had asked him how he passed the days he would have had no answer. He was doing a lot of thinking, but it all seemed to be circular. Over and over again, he reviewed the long list of skills, both vocational and avocational, that he had lost.

He had found a niche for himself within his social group of fellow dancers. It was one he held whether he could dance or not, so he had persisted in attending gatherings as an organizer while he wasn't a participant.

He had always been a loner at work, even though he got on well with the men. He was more interested in the work itself than he was in the small talk accompanying it. He couldn't really talk to the other men about his passionate interest in studying Balkan folk dance. However, they did understand his enthusiasm for the annual festival put on by the Slavic community—after all that was his heritage. As for the rest of the year, they could not be expected to understand. He went with the guys to sporting events or company barbecues, but he was not a family man and was not included in the more intimate social gatherings that had family as their focus. Still, he had held a place with these men of which he was proud. He could wield a hammer with the best of them—until today.

Before now, he had not let himself think about the possibility that he would not recover his strength and manual dexterity. He needed to think it through somehow. But he felt like he had just run into a brick wall. If only he hadn't dropped the teakettle, he would never have gone into the yard to see how well he could do. Damn the teakettle, anyway! How was he supposed to live? Stephen felt he needed an answer immediately. He kept thinking . . . and not answering the phone.

By the end of the week, there was no food in the house. Stephen tried to figure out what to do about that. There were several possibilities, but he could not seem to land on just the right one. It seemed that things had never looked bleaker than they did just now. He was faced with no food in the house, and no real desire to leave the house to get more. He knew that he needed to bathe and did not feel like he had the energy for that. He could not go out if he did not bathe—which he was not going to do today. Stephen thought he would just wait another day.

There was something else about tomorrow that was going to make shopping impossible, but Stephen could not remember what it was. He turned his limited powers of concentration to the new mystery. What was today, anyway? He had no idea. The paper would say. He went to the porch to bring in the paper and he was greeted by a stack of five rolled-up bundles. Stephen had to spread them all out and look for the one with the most recent date in order to discover that today was, indeed, Friday. That meant tomorrow would be Saturday. What was it about Saturday? Stephen could not remember, and he never wrote anything down on the kitchen calendar. Oh, well. Since the paper was already open, he leafed through it and found the answer to the Saturday mystery. Under local news, the paper announced that the annual spring dance festival was tomorrow at the university on the lawn outside the women's gymnasium from 1 to 4 p.m. Stephen sighed. He bathed, dressed, and went to the store.

COMMENTARY

Depression is a complicated emotional condition that comes in different forms and intensities. A major depression is a serious emotional illness marked by despondency and loss of interest in characteristic endeavors. Sometimes a major depression is caused by a biochemical imbalance in the brain. Other times it is the product of deep, unexpressed internal feelings, such as anger. This condition may persist for years and is accompanied by feelings of hopelessness, sadness, and fatigue. The afflicted person may move slowly and feel a great need to sleep, or may be troubled by restlessness. A severely depressed man, for instance, may lose all interest in sex. He may passively withdraw from all social contact. He may be unable to care for his home or his personal grooming. There seems to be no energy for a wide variety of feelings and activities. People suffering this profoundly disabling disease must have professional help.

It is important to distinguish this severe and prolonged emotional illness from Stephen's emotional *reaction*—his depressed state. Although sometimes encountered among the chronically ill, major depression is not a necessary or typical accompaniment of physical illness, as is Stephen's intermittent depression. The illness Stephen grapples with is stroke, not depression. His reaction to the loss that he has suffered we can call a *situational* depression. These depressions are more transient, and are reactions to stress.

Intermittent situational depression may have components of anxiety about the future, fear of getting sicker, frustration about limitations, and a sense of helplessness and dependency on people who may not be reliable. A situational depression may appear swiftly—as a reaction to trauma—or it may be more insidious—hidden behind a smiling face. Often, as in Stephen's case, a depressive episode is precipitated by the loss of a valued ability. We can expect these depressions to abate as the particular stress eases, or as the individual's adaptation and effective management of change increases, thereby affirming the value of his remaining capacities. Depression may recur when a sense of loss is rekindled and the stress is experienced anew.

We meet Stephen as his longing for the past collides with his weariness at daily living. His vivid dream of dancing at the festival tells us much about both his healthy and unhealthy responses to his loss of function. The dream provides respite from the daily struggle of his life. It reveals the longing for the happiness that dance has always brought him. For dance is to Stephen more than companionship; it is his form of creative self-expression and striving for excellence.

Stephen's unchanged desire for self-expression, his need to achieve quality—indeed excellence—in all he attempts are personality characteristics that may serve him well in his current life. How, then, does the dream signal emotional difficulties for Stephen? The danger signal is his idealized picture of the past. In his dream, life is sunny and perfect, and Stephen leading the line of dancers is the perfect Stephen. Remember, Stephen thinks that a year ago the dream was his complete reality. The truth, of course, is that it was just one moment in his reality. Such idealizations are always unreal. The "perfect Stephen" is his private *phantom psyche*, that is, the composite image of how life would be without any limitations. As long as Stephen allows this unrealistic, idealized image to exist unchallenged, his phantom psyche has the power to haunt him and belittle his current efforts.

Idealization of the past occurs even in the absence of illness, but illness seems to crystallize the past—when one had better physical function—into an image of perfection. It is not uncommon for people to think, "When I could walk unaided, I hadn't a care in the world." The nature of life, of course, is that there are worries, concerns, and frustrations. If Stephen loses sight of this practical reality, a reality faced by everyone, he runs the risk of being so self-critical, even of his successful efforts, that he can derive no pleasure, solace, or pride from his triumphs. He will begin to feel worthless.

These feelings of worthlessness are most apt to occur when there is some reminder of what has been lost and the patient begins to feel anxious. To some extent, these depressions are unavoidable. It helps to know, nevertheless, that they are to be expected, and that they have both realistic and unrealistic roots. Depressive moods generally abate as daily living routines are adapted to new limitations. The unrealistic components—the idealized past and exaggerated expectations of the future—tend to perpetuate depression. If Stephen were to remain trapped by his idea of a perfect past, he would inevitably turn his back on the present and not permit himself the opportunities for comfort available to him in his present life.

Even more troublesome for Stephen than the idealized past is the *adversary stance* he has taken toward his physical limitations. Stephen is used to being a competent fellow, a craftsman who has mastered a trade. He finds pleasure in precision and competition. Understandably, his experience of himself as a winner has led him to believe that he and his illness are opponents. The stroke is there to master. But Stephen is not a boxer in a ring, and there is no external opponent. The more he tries to beat the damage inflicted by his stroke, the more he beats himself up emotionally. After he drops the teakettle he feels very frightened. Instead of feeling relieved that he can still pick up the coffee mug, and with great effort clean up the spilled water, he saw the weakness in his arm as an enemy to be mastered. To assure himself that he was still master, he rushed off to fix the fence, and in doing so overtested his capabilities. Overtesting is a very common reaction to fear, and a very undermining one. It is a setup for failure and ensuing depression. Success is more likely to occur by taking small steps one at a time. In other words, attempt only what you can reasonably expect to achieve.

I am by no means suggesting that one cease struggling with new ways to handle difficulties imposed by illness. Nor that one give up customary satisfactions and habits as soon as a chronic disease is diagnosed. But one must realize that illness brings massive complications to living. To waste energy trying to annihilate an opponent, rather than learning how to live more fully, is one of the most commonly encountered emotional side effects of physical illness. To embrace an attitude that envisions illness only in terms of mastery or defeat invites tragedy, for it encourages thinking of oneself as a misfit or as a worthless human being—simply for being unable to do the impossible.

The adversary stance toward illness guarantees the patient will lose. It is important to realize that it was not Stephen's belief that he could conquer his first stroke that led to such a fine recovery. Whether Stephen realized it or not, it was his day-by-day diligence in trying to live life fully that helped him on his way.

Living more fully takes place one step at a time. If you have always loved gardening, you may not have to give it up entirely because of a physical disability. You may not be able to wield a rake and hoe, but you might be perfectly able to care for one flower bed, or to appreciate or help develop the gardening talents of another person. Stephen couldn't dance after the second stroke, but he still took pleasure in choosing the dances for others to perform. This approach may sound like a platitude—"Count your blessings" or some such empty phrase—but it really involves a crucial truth: appreciate what you have today—while you still have it. Stephen lost sight of living today when he encountered the frustrations of his second stroke.

Emotionally, this second stroke represented many things to Stephen. Rather than being rewarded for doing so well and trying so hard, it seemed he was being punished. He is likely to feel betrayed by fate, jealous of healthy people, and quite demoralized. Stephen would not be aware of all these negative feelings—characteristically he would believe he could muster his forces and conquer the stroke. But the negative feelings must have been there, below the surface; otherwise he would not have been so demoralized by such a minor setback as dropping the teakettle. When he could not change the weakness in his arm by willing that his arm be stronger, his feelings overwhelmed him and he became depressed. Stephen has to learn that fate can be neither controlled nor predicted. But what he can dramatically influence is his attitude about himself in the present. Stephen, as we know from his previous achievements, has many strengths, and his efforts at improving his life are very praiseworthy. At the moment he is temporarily overcome by frustration and anguish at the changes that time has wrought.

Depression is often triggered by an incident that underscores the patient's physical loss. The incident may seem trivial and may not be recognized by either patient or family as a precipitant of depression. This is because, on the surface, the triggering event bears little relationship to the degree of dread and panic that the patient feels internally. With Stephen it was dropping the kettle; with someone else it may be difficulty getting out of a bathtub.

Sometimes the reason for frustration and depression may be more obvious: for instance, a doctor's appointment that confirms an increase in symptoms. In any case, it is often true that neither patient, nor family, nor friends recognize the depth of anger and frustration accompanying the sense of disappointment.

The key here is what does the event, symptom, or change mean to the person? One person may be able to break crockery with impunity, but to another it may signal the end of one's days as a competent person. To a woman with many fine indoor plants, not being able to take care of them is a significant blow. A sensitive family member or friend who can care for the plants in the same way the patient would might shorten the period of despair. Someone else's way of doing it simply will not help. The patient must be consulted in the process so that she can remain actively involved.

Situational depressions do not disappear amid great fanfare, or in a dramatic way. They abate by degrees. The evidence of recovery is the return to habitual types of behavior and thought.

Many of us are inclined to approach depressed people with the suggestion "Cheer up. Everything's going to be all right." This does not help the patient, family, or friends. It merely makes an unrealistic and unwittingly cruel demand. The patient's physical reality is that something is not right, and will never be right again. Suggesting that it will also ignores the family's emotional stress of trying to quickly adapt to major changes in life circumstances. Unlike empty reassurances, genuine loving care will be enormously helpful to patients. There are a number of ways helpers can demonstrate their caring.

In many ways, the key is to continue treating the patient as a "normal" person. He is a normal person who happens to have an illness. If the patient is present, talk to him, not about him. Continuation of good grooming is a must for patient morale. If the patient is physically able, the grooming tasks are his domain. When he is unable, caretakers need to assume this responsibility—a good bed-bath is refreshing. If the patient's daily chore has been to set the table, encourage him to continue doing so. The critical issue is that there be a good match between physical ability and expectations of activity. A bedridden family member may be a most capable arithmetic tutor, and may enjoy being one even if the sessions are a few minutes at a time. The one major restriction in establishing goals is that no large demands should be imposed on the patient. Helping a child with math homework may be fine. However, demanding that the patient prepare the income tax returns is both unrealistic and cruel.

Patients like Stephen, who are living alone, require a certain kind of monitoring from helpers. Aside from calling and helping as necessary with chores, friends should take the responsibility of dropping by the patient's home if there is any break in customary contact. Stephen would probably have answered the doorbell even if he didn't answer the phone, and this small activity would have helped him to regain a more healthy perspective about his condition. In extreme cases, where there is no response from the patient and where household neglect is evident, friends should ask the police to make a safety check.

Many things are capable of boosting morale, including an affectionate pet. For the single person this can be especially important, but for anyone a pet's demands for care and its unquestioning affection can be very heartening.

For all patients, open recognition of their difficult struggle is helpful. This combined with overt signs of affection, and the expectation that they can reciprocate, is revitalizing to a depressed person. The patient must also realize that his smile, or thank you, or quiet recognition of help given is important for his emotional recovery.

There are times when reciprocity cannot exist, either because the patient is too depressed or the family is too discouraged. Here is when friends can be most helpful. They can provide respite for the family as well as novelty for the patient. A friend can do a real service by visiting with the patient while the caretaker has some time alone.

The end result of all helpful and caring approaches is that patients and their families will come to truly feel that the patient and his illness are not one in the same thing.

CHAPTER SIX

RENEWAL

Crisp morning sun awakened Susan. Even before she moved, she enjoyed the tranquility that a good night's sleep always granted her. She liked to lie in bed for a few minutes and savor the first mood of the day—provided that it was a good one. Today felt like a good day—there was an air of promise about it. Susan had learned not to spoil anticipation of good things by the everpresent need to attend to the negatives in her life. Therefore she simply enjoyed the coziness of the comforter and the mattress heater that kept her warm and relatively pain-free during the night.

At age 55, Susan had a keen intelligence, a lively interest in other people, many projects for diversion, and an advanced case of arthritis. This last meant pain, loss of mobility, loss of her old self-image as a spry, strong woman, and much more confinement than she had been comfortable with until recently. It was the pain, though, that had completely demoralized her and could still do so, at times. She hated to risk disturbing this morning's sense of well-being by inducing pain through the simplest of movements. Her life had not been a bed of roses, certainly, and she could accept that, but she still dreaded the days that became a bed of thorns.

This day had begun rather nicely, but she would have to find out what she would be dealing with to know whether the day's plans stood a chance of materializing. She had a lunch date with a friend whom she really looked forward to seeing. These days pain often called for the restructuring of plans, but she did not let go of anything she did not have to that might bring her pleasure.

Basically, Susan was a highly realistic woman. Over the years her fundamental realism made her understand and finally accept that she was able to do less and less. She had also come to realize that she need not stop growing as a person because of her illness. She knew that she had to coexist with pain and physical limitation, and not let it always dominate her life or self-definition. It had taken her long years to really understand this. Of course, it was not always possible to maintain this perspective, but she kept coming back to it.

Susan's first flash of pain was expected. Tentatively she began to ease herself from the bed. The pain that shot through her hip joints was fiery and penetrating. But even as her eyes teared unavoidably, she felt that at some level she was calmer than she used to be—she didn't have that intense dread of pain that she used to experience. She hated the pain while it lasted because it drained her of energy she would like to have spent in other ways. But at this point she knew she was a survivor, and she could draw sustenance from that self-awareness. To know that she could make it through another day, regardless of what it entailed, was an enormous improvement over not wanting to live another day. Now she was able to give herself credit for each day's struggle, and to look for ways she could minimize the day's emotional toil for herself and for those who cared about her.

Susan was Susan, first and foremost. These days she was seldom just a woman with crippling arthritis. This awareness was the result of a long, tumultuous, sometimes tedious process to continue being.

Susan had always been a determined, high-spirited person. It had simply never crossed her mind as a newlywed in her 20s that life could be anything but terrific. It had proved something less than terrific when in her early 30s she found she had arthritis. This had not been altogether surprising since there was plenty of arthritis on her father's side of the family. In fact, Susan had always admired how uncomplaining her father seemed to be as he went to work on days when he was in pain. In the early days, Susan felt she lived up to her family's stoical standards—she had not complained either. Of course, she'd had no idea how bad the pain could really be.

She was also to learn about emotional pain with the death of her husband. Not quite 40, he had been a prosperous young attorney when he died. Fortunately for Susan, her less prosperous, but very practical parents had talked her husband into purchasing life and health insurance when Susan and her husband were in their 20s. Susan had been overwhelmed with grief, but at least she did not have to face the additional burden of poverty. She had felt so uncharacteristically blue and unproductive, however, that she sought counseling. And this proved very helpful.

Nevertheless, she'd experienced increasing physical pain and difficulty moving around, and, noticing this, her therapist had suggested another visit to the doctor. Susan knew that when people are in mourning it is not unusual for them to experience physical problems. However, both she and her therapist suspected that her increased physical discomfort could not simply be explained by the added stress of widowhood. Her physician had confirmed their suspicions— the arthritis had definitely advanced. Susan was given pain killers and anti-inflammatory medication. Physically she had felt much better, but emotionally she was floundering. How was she to deal with all of this?

Susan had realized she was cutting herself off from friends—or at least from the healthy ones or married ones of whom she felt jealous. She'd felt bitterly disappointed with life and with herself. She'd grow angry over the smallest things. Both she and her therapist had felt it was time to do something about Susan's increasing isolation. In truth, Susan had missed all her social contacts. She'd even missed all the pleasant contact with her deceased husband's business associates. The people from his office—a few of the secretaries in particular—had stayed in touch with her. Susan was trained as a paralegal assistant, so when she heard via the grapevine that there was an opening for a paralegal in a familiar law firm working for people she liked, she'd applied for the job.

For an instant, when she put the application in the mail, Susan had felt like herself again. It was the first inkling of inner peace she had had in some time. She and her therapist had tried to anticipate the relative advantages of getting or not getting the job. Susan had felt well prepared for either outcome. As quickly as the job was offered to her, she'd accepted.

She had loved having a place to go each day. She liked being a cog in the wheels of the large firm. But hour after hour of research and formulating documents had left Susan in extreme physical discomfort. Over time, the discomfort became intense pain. Susan had to resign, and soon lapsed into another depression. She was worthless after all—she could not keep up with the demands of daily living. The only benefit of her sojourn in the work world was renewed, active friendships. That thought had pleased her until she undid all the good feelings by telling herself that the people in the office would soon forget her now that she was not there every day. Her therapist had reminded her that she could call the friends, but Susan had resisted this idea. She, after all, was the one who felt crummy—why should she have to do the calling? For a while she had not called anyone. Her friends had tried to keep in touch, but Susan had felt she had nothing to say to them that they'd want to hear.

Susan's husband had died when she was 35. It had taken her two years to build up the courage to try working. The disappointment about giving up the job had precipitated a depression that lasted two more years. Then a shocking thing happened. Susan's arthritis, which had responded to medical treatment and which had not seemed to be getting worse at an alarming rate, suddenly became so much worse that she was in effect confined to bed. Her life had been consumed with pain. There seemed to be no Susan—only an engulfing pain. She had been so depleted physically that she had not even felt depressed; just disinterested and removed from everything except the searing pain in her joints.

Finally, Susan's practical side had taken command. There had to be something to do about the pain, and she began to dedicate all her available energy to defeating it. So she obtained various heating appliances; she took a course on pain management, learning about relaxation and self-hypnosis; she investigated biofeedback, acupuncture, vitamin therapy. She and her doctor experimented with various medications and dosages. Once more, Susan's days felt busy, but she had barely been able to move a muscle without being aware that she had not won the battle with pain. Again, Susan felt discouraged and had despaired of ever feeling whole again. That was a truly terrifying thought, and she had struggled for years to keep it hidden from herself. But the facts were that she was a widow faced with increasing pain and declining ability to get about as she wished.

Looking back, Susan could remember how scared she was. But there had also been that small part of her that persisted in seeing beyond fear and pain, that continued to look outward, and to have concern for other people. And a small but persistent inner voice told her over and over again that she was fighting with herself unnecessarily.

She had not even understood what she meant by that the first time the idea came to her. She knew she could not just give up—so didn't that mean she had to fight something? "Try giving yourself credit for what you can do, rather than berating yourself for what you cannot," the inner voice had responded. She knew she had heard that at home when her mother would console her father. Really, it was a warm, comforting, and sensible thought. But it had taken her years to feel sustained by it.

Somewhere around age 45, Susan began to make this idea a living principal. She saw time running out for other people, and she didn't want it running out for her. So she made some new resolutions. First, somehow, she was going to make life easier for herself. She wasn't sure what more she could do physically, but she did know she had to stop accusing herself of failure. Maybe she could be nicer to herself somehow.

A good friend had once advised Susan to celebrate during the times she felt low.

"Do what?" had been Susan's reply.

"Celebrate. You don't need it when everything feels fine. But indulge yourself when you feel rotten."

Susan had dismissed this as silly at first, but later she saw how it could fit in with her resolve to treat herself better.

She "celebrated" by redecorating her bedroom. The freshly painted room with rose accents was enormously pleasing to her. Her one problem with the large bedroom was the distance between her bed and bathroom. Susan began to wonder about aids to help her with that trek. She already had a walker. In the past she had seen this walker as a symbol of failure to meet a personally set goal of recovery. Now she was wondering if the walker were sufficient. For some reason, she remembered the sturdy ballet bars on which she had exercised as a child. What if she put such a rail along the wall between the bed and the bathroom? The walker could get her to the wall, then it would be up to her and the rail. She liked the idea, both because it was a change and because it was a way of dividing a chore into two manageable pieces— the completion of each part might make the whole task easier and more satisfying.

Before long, Susan had transformed her bedroom into an interesting combination boudoir and gymnasium: ballet bar on the wall, exercycle in the corner, swim gear on a shelf near the bike. By her bed she had a personally designed bedstand with sliding trays containing pens, pads of paper, books, medications, and snacks. The phone was easily accessible. To Susan, the overall effect was both cheerful and satisfying. She could be productive without having to move much on days when she really could not. And on days when she could do a little better, she had every available contrivance to assist her. She even got a rubber cover for the overflow drain on her tub so that she could get four extra inches of hot water to soak in. A real inspiration was to convert her hand-powered carpet sweeper into an exercise tool. She could sit on the edge of her bed and work the light-weight sweeper back and forth to improve flexibility in her shoulders and elbows. She was so enthused about the ballet bars that she decided to install them in other places around the house.

Susan had learned to recognize that creative use of ballet bars, carpetsweepers, or other aids was an important accomplishment—not a sign of failure. She grew to realize that she would never meet all her standards for recovery, and that noticing progress, even when that meant maintaining the status quo, was more important. Unrealistic standards had for too long deprived her of a current existence, whereas recognizing progress affirmed her life-oriented strivings.

A second resolution was more difficult to carry out—to enrich her social contacts. She didn't want to lose contact with people she cared about, and she wanted to rekindle some old friendships—and maybe make some new ones. For nearly ten years she had felt that the burden of communicating was on her friends. But the one exception had always been the Christmas cards and notes she wrote. When she had to, she hired someone to address the envelopes, but she would try to write a card a day, from October on. This way she still knew where people lived and something about their lives. She could still remember sitting in bed, intermittently resting her hands on a heating pad, and how much satisfaction she felt with the slow, painstaking completion of each note. Those were almost happy feelings. And, of course, she felt most happy when her greetings were returned, for any validation of her worthiness as a friend had become very important to Susan.

Making a phone call, however, was far more frightening. After all, the payoff was immediate—and uncertain. She couldn't be sure how the person she called would respond. And whatever the response, she felt so exposed. There is simply no facesaving on the telephone. At first, calls were really difficult, and sometimes her fears of rejection were borne out. But the exhilarating response from some of her friends made all of her efforts worthwhile.

Pain brought Susan's thoughts back to the present. It was truly going to be a difficult day. She succeeded in placing her feet on the floor, and with effort pulled herself up with the walker. She made it to the bars. Every step was agonizing, but she persisted in moving slowly back and forth along that wall until she had some degree of flexibility. She had several hours to get ready for her lunch date. This would ordinarily mean bathing, dressing, and becoming limber enough to walk with the support of the walker. But gauging the pain, she knew she was not going out of the house today. She would call Linda and ask her to bring in sandwiches from the deli instead. Linda would understand.

Linda had been one of the friends Susan had reclaimed several years after the illness had changed her life. Linda had originally fled from their relationship, but Susan thought enough of her to wish to continue the contact. Though in time Linda turned out to be one of Susan's most obliging friends, she was also one of her most frightened. Linda's initial comment about the bedroom had been "My God, you've built yourself a hospital room."

Linda's remark about the bedroom typified the difficulty she had with Susan's chronic illness. In an unenlightened but direct way, she commented on her disappointment that Susan was not able to continue living as if there were no illness. Beneath the disappointment was an active fear that Susan's fate might become her own.

Susan knew of her friend's fear, and was therefore especially delighted that Linda tried so hard to be helpful to her. When Susan finally made the decision not to fight the disease, but to live life more fully, she began redoing her house. Unlike Linda's fearful reaction, Susan knew that whatever she could do to ease her life—from ballet bars to inexpensive mail-order devices—would automatically improve its quality. And Susan's concern was with the quality of her life. She had absolutely no need to tire herself out just to impress the neighbors or friends. Her energy was hers to use as she saw fit, and she conserved it in order to be able to focus it on the people and activities that were meaningful to her.

Lunch was good. Susan truly enjoyed Linda's company. They worked together volunteering some time at the local senior center. Susan had taken on a task that could be done primarily at home, while Linda ran errands for two elderly women one day a week. They had a good long talk, and by the time Linda left, Susan was ready for a rest. She and her friend David were going to try a matinee tomorrow, if all went well.

Linda was not the only friend she had succeeded in retrieving from the past. A close college friend, David, after several years of silence and a painful divorce, eventually got back in touch with her. When David's job moved him within 30 miles of her town, he began to drop around occasionally. They discovered that they still enjoyed one another's company, and an easy, frank manner developed between them. David would make a few social pleasantries, and Susan would respond in kind. Then he began asking what he could do to help her.

"Is there anything that needs fixing, Susan?"

Susan was a very organized person and always had a list of a zillion items in need of repair. Her friend, with good humor, tackled what he could. Susan felt it was significant that she didn't have to ask for help before David realized she might need some.

One day, rather routinely, David had again asked what needed fixing.

"I do."

David had been shocked—dismayed to hear her voice such a low opinion of herself. "What do you mean? You're not a selfish or malicious person. There are lots of people who don't need physical help who need fixing much more than you ever could. "

Susan was taken aback. Apparently part of her was still not ready to relinquish the idea that she was damaged. She still had trouble separating her sense of self-worth from the physical damage, dependency, and loneliness she struggled with. What was wonderful to her was that David could separate her value from her problems, and it was helpful to have a friend who could be that kind of mirror for her.

By noon the next day Susan was able to get around rather comfortably. She dressed to go out with David. Her hands seemed to be the worst of it today, but she had been acquiring clothes over the years that required little from her fingers. The dress looked nice, and her outfit needed only a necklace. She selected the one she wanted and realized right away she would be unable to fasten it herself. So today David's query about whether she needed help would get a simple answer—"Only my necklace, please." And Susan smiled as she thought of the mundane but terribly important domesticity of this request.

She and David had no future plans. He had tried to formalize their relationship on several occasions, but Susan had rejected the idea of marriage. At first she had told herself that she still felt too much grief for her deceased husband; then that David was still too close to his divorce. But her most persistent and unspoken reason was that she had always been afraid of being a burden, imposing her restrictions on David. Along with the many other things that had changed in her outlook, today Susan knew she would not be an imposition. She and David were responsible adults who knew what they wanted and what they could handle. "Who knows," she said to herself. "If David doesn't bring it up himself, perhaps I'll pop the question again soon."

COMMENTARY

Renewal is the last stage of a long and uneven process of emotional growth, and in it we can see elements of all the other stages that we've explored. Renewal is the rediscovery of valued aspects of yourself that make it possible to feel content in many circumstances, and to feel real joy in those moments of rapport with another or with yourself.

Throughout the emotional process accompanying chronic physical illness, you have confronted terror, loss, rage—every variety of emotional pain. Renewal begins to take place and is strengthened every time you are able to face fear of the unknown and pain related to loss. By facing these dreads, you can learn that they are not so overwhelming that all direction in your life is lost.

In many ways, renewal is the result of finding yourself once again. A self in new circumstances, with more constraints to handle, but with the tools to continue in life regardless of the recurring sense that life has changed too radically to be recognizable.

What is the essence of renewal? How can you find yourself when so much has been lost? The usual answers of "give it time" or "you've just got to adjust" miss the most vital aspect of this phase. Renewal is not static, nor is it passive. It is a dynamic attitude toward illness, born of all the past struggles with the disease. You set and reset your priorities in such a way that the capacities affected by illness no longer define you.

Finding yourself is always a journey. Under these circumstances there are points of the journey that seem catastrophic. In fact, the physical reality is often devastating. Those who reach renewal have discovered something beyond physical constraint. What they have found is the ability to appreciate moments of respite from the struggle, to savor everyday events, and to recognize how much they can influence their own lives.

In the process of renewal, "Why me?" yields to "Why not me?" and then to "Who do I choose to be?" Not what does my illness make me, but who can I be, given my limitations and the understanding that I may be physically disabled without being emotionally handicapped. There is nothing apologetic about renewal. It is an ever-changing, alert awareness of the possibilities of today.

A hallmark of renewal is the hard-won ability to separate yourself from your illness. How do we see this in Susan? After years of depression Susan began to take enough risks that she could reexperience life as having some of the promise she had valued in her optimistic 20s. The Susan we meet is seasoned and scarred, but not lost. She never ignores her illness; she is always aware of her real physical limitations. But whenever she can, she makes other current experiences the focus of her life. Thus, she enjoys the comfortable sensations of waking, warm and relaxed, even though she knows pain will follow. When she finds she can't go out, she still focuses on the pleasures of visiting with her friends, rather than on her limitations. She uses part of her available energy to help other people—she is actively engaged with living.

The creative adaptation to illness is another essential characteristic of renewal. Susan demonstrated a highly constructive and creative reaction to her immobility and severe pain. She designed her bedroom in such a way that it was a pleasing and safe room for her. She did not see the use of aids as giving up or feeling sorry for herself. Quite the reverse, she saw them as providing the means to more important ends—as a way to conserve energy so that she could be with friends and have some diversion from the toil of living.

We also see in Susan a third foundation of renewal. Over the years she was able to experience less concern about the future. She has few future-oriented anxieties, and is, in contrast, heavily invested in today and what it can bring her. Not in today and what it will do to her, but in what she can make happen for herself that is fulfilling. This attitude is possible to the extent that the turmoil of the earlier stages has resulted in a reduced dread of the unknown.

If we fear the future we rob ourselves of today. Paradoxically, those of us who face our vulnerability over and over again and realize how easily health can fragment eventually experience less dread and increase our potential for present satisfaction. In doing this, Susan is not pretending there are no problems, but much of the time she is not caught in the fearsome trap of dreading each day's passage.

During the early emotional stages people often suffer from extreme guilt about their illnesses. The guilt doesn't serve a constructive purpose, and may add enough stress that certain conditions worsen. The renewed person wastes little energy on feeling guilty about the disease and reserves guilt for when it is deserved—when you mistreat another person, for instance.

Susan, like many of us, was fearful that she would be a burden to her friends. This is really another way of feeling guilty about having to ask for help. Now she was able to accept help from David, and to even ask for it from trusted friends—without shame.

Disappointment in other people, and jealousy of them, is a natural reaction to chronic illness. These feelings are not always expressed overtly, but may cause you to feel unworthy. Susan suffered from this self-perception, and kept herself socially isolated during times when she was much more physically capable than when we meet her. Only when she recognized how self-perpetuating and isolating her depression was did she make active use of her therapist's guidance and begin to take social risks again. Signs of Susan's increasing freedom from guilt and jealousy include her ability to reach out to others, risking rejection.

Like all other phases of emotional recovery, renewal is a dynamic state. You do not simply reach the point of renewal and stay put—there are bound to be lapses. Susan's most striking lapse is evident in her self-disparaging remark that she needed to be fixed. At that point, her focus had shifted from her own potential to the imagined potential of other people. Nevertheless she was able to accept both David's criticism and assistance. That she can even contemplate a more serious and lasting relationship shows us that she had not really lost her attitude of self-acceptance.

Like others struggling for renewal, Susan is no stranger to a thought process something like this: I am a person who happens to have an illness. I can no longer do certain things. More importantly, I am a person who can acknowledge what my feelings are about myself and my physical predicament. I can be sad and upset when it is appropriate. I continue with as much positive feeling and activity in my life as I can. I strive not to judge myself too harshly. I accept the limitations of others while continuing to flexibly adapt to my own changing circumstances. I have seen the cost to me of holding on to anger, bitterness, and jealousy. I have the power to choose not to continue these feelings. I must recognize my own emotional and physical vulnerability and let that be acceptable. I do not give up on myself. I trust I will continue to do what I can with what I have today, so that tomorrow—should those abilities be lost to me—I will have few regrets about the way I lived today. Any time you find yourself thinking along these lines, you are doing very well emotionally. You deserve applause for being able-hearted.

Indeed, part of being able-hearted is being able to separate and appreciate the individual experiences of each day, so that days are not simply mass impressions. When you do this, you will find many reasons to be satisfied with what the day has been; you may see ways in which to try doing similar tasks differently and more adaptively; and, you will perceive the potential of tomorrow without needing to dictate precisely what tomorrow will be. This last point is critical. Based on today's positive experiences of yourself—however fleeting—there is hope that tomorrow can be taken in stride. And you will try to engage with and participate in whatever opportunities are inherent in that day. Some of these will merely occur, and may feel more like burdens than opportunities. Some of these will be actively created by you. The essential element is a sense of potential. It is an internal potential which we can act on at least part of the time. It combines fortitude, desire, self-acceptance, and whimsy.

Allow your intent, curiosity, and determination to coexist with uncertainty be the basis of your self-definition, and forgive yourself for what you are unable to do. The exquisite ability to be connected to yourself, others, and to your environment outweighs the physical limitations on doing. You are not just what you do. You are a complete person, and you are entitled to all the complexities, sorrows, and joys of being able-hearted.

CHAPTER SEVEN

HELPING.

So far this book has focused on those who have a chronic illness or disability. This chapter is for those who are their helpers. It is especially for the family members and close friends who are called upon to meet the emotional challenges of those they care for who are afflicted with a chronic illness.

In the lives of my patients, the stress of chronic illness on family and friends is very clear. Some, when confronted with the hard reality of an unwanted and unforeseen illness, flee the situation. Some blame the patient or blame themselves. This prevents successful coping. Some cannot change the relationships and patterns of activities that were functional before the illness or disability occurred, and which are no longer useful.

But many family members and friends find new strengths in themselves and in those they care for. They construct new ways of finding meaning and pleasure in their relationships. Like those with chronic illness who have passed through the stages to self-renewal and have found new ways to achieve success and satisfaction, caregivers must also pass through often difficult stages to find their own renewal.

This chapter will comment on the roles of the caregiver at each of the stages of chronic illness. It will then outline some specific personal concerns for caregivers.

There are two postures that need to be avoided. You should not try to be a hero. Nor should you see yourself as a martyr.

The hero posture imagines that through superhuman, almost magical effort, the overwhelming challenge of chronic illness can be overcome. The triumph of the hero will be recognized and applauded by all, and everyone will live happily ever after.

Chronic illness does not respond to heroics. By definition it is not going to be vanquished. Those who try to be hero helpers are always disappointed, and they do not provide the long-term, consistent helping relationship that is needed.

The martyr posture imagines that cruel fate has visited this terrible calamity upon the helper who must suffer visibly so that the martyr's woes are recognized and pitied by all.

Chronic illness does not respond to lamentations and martyr helpers are always disappointed. More importantly, they cannot provide the long-term, consistent helping relationship that is needed. It is often useful to think of yourself as a pioneer in a strange land. Despite unknown terrors and hazards, in the face of daunting difficulties and frustrations, you keep moving on into uncharted territory, seeking the understanding, strength, and mastery that will allow successful living in a new land.

The successful pioneers penetrated the unknown to build satisfying new lives. The pioneer helper must do the same in the unexplored territory of the chronic illness of a family member or friend. While heroes and martyrs are lonely callings, pioneers seldom strike out alone. They depend upon the support of many other people. To be a successful pioneer helper, you will often need to call upon others—other family members, friends, support groups, and professionals.

The most important idea in this chapter is this: The physical realities of illness or disability do not define the essence of a human being. A person with chronic physical limitations has values, goals, behaviors, beliefs, attitudes, feelings, capabilities, creativity, passions, and personality that make up the essence of that person.

You as a helper are also a person with values, goals, behaviors, beliefs, attitudes, feelings, capabilities, creativity, passions, and personality. You cannot be defined by the chronic physical limitations of the person you are helping.

Both of your identities are defined independently of any illness or physical disability. Because of this, your relationship before the illness or disability and your relationship after the illness or disability should be far more similar than different. A broken arm would not change a relationship because it would clearly not change the essence of the personality.

The more serious chronic illnesses and disabilities bring about many changes. However, they do not change the core relationship that existed before the onset of the illness or disability.

Here is an overview of key elements in mastering unavoidable changes.

1. You must recognize and understand the factual nature of reality as quickly as you can, without allowing yourself to be overwhelmed. Be open to the true state of affairs.

2. From the beginning take responsibility for your own reactions and responses to the situation. Your reactions to the unpleasantness of the illness must not carry over and affect your responses to the person who is ill.

3. Avoidance of the reality of the illness is an easy, common, and sometimes necessary response to a chronic disability. But the consequences of avoidance are the reinforcement of fear, alienation, and isolation. Avoidance seems to bring relief from the uncertainty and pain, but it soon produces guilt and inhibits useful action.

4. Communicate freely and often with many others. Talk to friends, family, medical personnel, spiritual advisers, and of course, the patient. Don't be afraid to air your fears and concerns. Don't hesitate to ask for understanding and support. Open and frequent communication is part of the healing process, and is necessary to everyone involved. Communication shores up emotional strength in times of high stress.

5. Look at all parts of life. Caring for a loved one who is suffering often puts the focus on the bad side of life. Troubles seem to be all that there are. But life has many facets. Amidst the troubles there are always good things occurring. Look for them.

6. The uncertainties and difficulties of change will lead to mistakes and errors. Your limitations and weaknesses will seem to be more stark than ever. You cannot allow yourself to be weighed down by the inevitable mishaps that will occur. You must treat your own mistakes and limitations gently. Accept them and move on. Learn from them. Treat yourself with understanding so that you have the peace of mind and the energy that will help you to be a competent caregiver.

7. Develop an understanding of how the medical system works. Ask questions and investigate. The current environment, with its concern over the costs of medical

care, often results in patients receiving less medical care than was given in the past. Hospital stays may be cut short. The patient will often need the services of visiting nurses, physical therapists, and other professionals to come to the home. Family, friends, church groups, or other groups are often needed to assist with household duties, personal care requirements, and even nursing-type activities. Be sure that you understand how the doctor and the hospital intend to handle the treatment and the discharge of the patient. Find out what the patient will need when released from the hospital. Then make plans to accommodate the needs that will arise. Seek out the discharge planning social worker to help.

8. Check yourself each day. Ask yourself questions such as, "Am I getting enough to eat, enough sleep? Am I making opportunities to relieve my own stress? Do I have the information I need to take care of the ill person today? Have I adjusted satisfactorily to the new reality that now affects our lives and our relationship?" If your responses to this self-examination do not feel right, then it is time to consult with someone who can help. This may be a medical practitioner, a counselor, a clergy person, a wise family member, or a trusted friend. You cannot be an effective caregiver if your own physical and emotional life is not attended to.

9. Avoid guilt and self-reproach. Helpers often blame themselves for the illness that has afflicted the one they care for. That is neither useful nor realistic. Helpers may blame the patient—"If you had only done as I told you, this wouldn't have happened." This, too, is neither useful nor realistic.

This book has outlined six stages of chronic physical illness. At each stage there are specific roles and actions that helpers need to take.

CRISIS

In the acute crisis stage of illness the patient seldom has the capability for extensive interaction with helpers. Friends and family are caught between waiting for more medical information and the pressures of daily life, a life that must now be managed without the participation of the patient. However, it is a time for helpers to prepare themselves. They need to gain as much understanding as possible of the reality of the situation. They need to take steps to prepare for the time when the patient's illness has moved beyond the acute crisis stage. Preparations must be made for the changes that are going to occur.

The chapter on crisis gives much attention to the helpers and their responses. Rather than repeat the insights and information given there, you should reread this chapter from the helper's perspective.

ISOLATION

In this stage patients often become isolated from the normal relationships that have sustained them in their pre-illness lives. This is a time when frequent and open communication is essential. Helpers must make a conscious, active effort to maintain communications.

The commentary at the end of this chapter gives specific assistance in understanding the kinds of communication that are needed.

A major difficulty for those who are just coming to realize the nature of their disability is asking for help. Most of us are trained from infancy to be independent; not asking for help is often a sign of maturity. It is very difficult to overcome this conditioning and learn to ask for help. There are mental conflicts about the meaning of dependence and independence. We often fail to see that asking for help is a tool to promote independence.

Helpers, through their actions, can either facilitate or make impossible the patient's ability to ask for help. Helpers can and must play a major part in overcoming the reluctance to ask for help. During the isolation stage it is often desirable to comment to the ill person, "You seem to need something." This kind of inquiry indicates the helper's willingness to assist without assuming to know what the patient needs. This must be done cheerfully and in a way that implies no feeling of imposition or obligation on the part of the helper. It is easier to ask a person for help if that person has demonstrated a willingness to pitch in without being asked, and without complaining.

Learning to ask for needed help is a necessary part of coming to terms with a chronic disability. And one of the most important tasks for helpers is to be responsive to the patient's task of learning and practicing to ask for help.

ANGER

Anger is a natural response to chronic illness and disability. It is a stage that puts great stress on helping relationships. The patient's anger is often directed inward. But often enough it can erupt as anger toward friends, family, medical personnel, and others with whom the patient is in regular contact.

All of us, when we are tired or stressed, can lash out in anger at those we love. Those with chronic illness, dealing with rage, have even more provocation to express their anger to those around them. This is hardly a comfortable or pleasant situation for helpers. However, it is a stage through which the patient must pass. Anger is best answered with understanding and caring. It is not helpful to respond to anger with more anger.

Anger should be viewed as an outpouring of energy. It can often be rechanneled, becoming an outflow of positive energy. Just as the patient's anger might be focused usefully on difficult physical therapy, the helper's anger might be focused usefully on taking care of daily living activities, making necessary phone calls, seeking information from medical personnel, and so forth. By expending the energy on productive activities it is often possible to reduce the level of anger.

Anger is often expressed inwardly as anger at oneself. This can be very debilitating to patients. Helpers must watch carefully for indications that the patient is directing anger inward, and then seek to bring the anger out into the open so that it can be rechanneled or mitigated. Helpers must also be alert to signs of depression in themselves.

In the case of anger which cannot be dealt with, it is often useful to get the assistance of a mental-health specialist. Even the most dedicated helper cannot cope with every problem.

RECONSTRUCTION

In the reconstruction stage the patient begins to rebuild emotional strength. It is often a time when changes in lifestyle must be made, and when it is possible to undertake new activities to replace those that can no longer be handled.

Helpers must be willing to accept the changes. After a period during which the helper often had to take the primary responsibility for decisions, the patient is now ready to take back responsibility for much of his own life. Sometimes it is difficult for the helper to switch from being the decision-maker to playing a supporting role. The story of Peter and Lorraine illustrates some of the issues that helpers face during reconstruction.

Helpers have an important role to play in helping patients learn to live each day. They must also incorporate that philosophy into their own lives. Life is not something that happens later. It is a process of positives and negatives that is going on right now. Planning only for future pleasures is not a constructive way to live. With a chronic illness or disability it is very important to capture pleasure and satisfaction now. Of course, not every moment of any life can be all pleasure and satisfaction. But both helper and patient will benefit from acknowledging the simple pleasures and moments of joy in each day.

INTERMITTENT DEPRESSION

Chronic illness, disability, old age—any situation in which our capabilities have been lessened—can occasion bouts of depression. Depression is a part of life. It is not a moral failing.

Severe depression is a clinical condition that needs the attention of professionals. Signs of grave depression include trouble sleeping, weight gain or weight loss, feelings of hopelessness or worthlessness, unrelenting irritability, loss of interest in people, including the self, and the wish to die.

Helpers must be prepared to deal with the less serious intermittent depression faced by the patient or that they themselves face.

There are several things that helpers can do. It is important to keep the patient and the illness separate, and emphasize that you value the patient as a person—that you value your relationship with the patient.

Communication is essential during this stage. There needs to be conscious, consistent effort given to maintain communications. Depressed people often do not want to talk. They lapse into discouraged silence. Helpers can work to build and maintain conversation. One can begin with news of the family, or neighborhood, or whatever. Draw out the patient by asking for reactions and opinions. Don't be surprised if these are sour and short in the beginning. Persistence and determination should eventually engage the patient and create the communication that can help draw the patient out of a depressed state.

It is useful for helpers to recognize that the patient's depression usually has a compelling cause. Coping with disability is a struggle that often seems to produce no results. Express your recognition of the validity of the struggle, and the depression that it can produce. Express affection. Be responsive. Helpers may find that their own depression makes it impossible to be emotionally responsive in the relationship. If this occurs, helpers need to seek help for themselves.

Depression is not an easy stage for helpers. Sometimes it is necessary to enlist others to provide the primary helper with time to recharge. By recognizing that intermittent depression is likely to occur, helpers can be better prepared to cope with it and live through it to the next stage.

RENEWAL

Renewal is the easiest stage for helpers. In this stage, the patient is able to find contentment and satisfaction. It is easier to ask for help. The patient has learned how to live each day, and to find joy and satisfaction in what can be done, rather than to dwell on what cannot be done.

The helper and the patient can develop an easy and comfortable relationship in which each accepts the reality of the handicap, but knows that it does not define the person or the relationship.

Helpers need to recognize when renewal is occurring. At this stage it is often necessary to back off and give the patient more opportunity for personal growth and achievement. The helper who continues to want to do everything and make all the decisions can retard or kill renewal. The patient is now able to manage his or her own life much more completely than before. Of course, help will still be needed, but it can be given and received with much less fuss and concern than in previous stages.

Renewal is the stage that rewards patients and helpers for growing through the other stages.

It is well to keep in mind that these stages do not occur in a straight line going in one direction. The path is more like a spiral in which stages are revisited. After renewal a new crisis may occur. Some setback in capability can easily trigger a bout of depression.

Helpers should expect to revisit various stages. Like a spiral that goes upward, the passage through the stages will be different each time. In particular, the skills and experience that the helper gained the first time around will make the next occurrence easier to handle. Having seen a relationship through the darkest stages and come through to renewal, it is easier to believe that the relationship will once again survive to another time of renewal.

To be a good helper, you need to understand yourself. Consider the following questions. They will help you to know your own strengths and weaknesses better.

1. How open, direct, and honest was your communication and relationship with the patient prior to the illness or disability?

2. Have you and the patient faced very difficult challenges before? What strengths did you call upon then? What did you learn from that experience?

3. Do you rely on others to handle the really difficult or frightening issues that arise? Do you back away from situations that might be stressful or frustrating? Or are you able to cope with tough times?

4. Is the patient your only trusted support person? Or are there others you can lean on in a time of stress?

5. Have you learned how to grieve? Have you been able to turn to others when you need help in handling grief-producing situations?

6. Have you been comfortable in dealing with the "public"—the many outsiders who play a role in your life and the patient's life? Or have you depended upon the patient to be the intermediary between you and other people?

7. Who has taken the primary responsibility for maintaining the relationship between you and the patient?

With illness, we are dealing with an unwelcome and uninvited reality. The questions above deal with important aspects of relationships. Facing reality means being realistic about your own experiences, capabilities, and comfort in dealing with others.

You must also be realistic about your relationships with yourself, if you are to be an effective helper. These are questions that will help you think about yourself.

1. What are the things you like best about yourself? What do you consider your strengths to be?

2. What are the things you like least about yourself? What do you consider your weaknesses to be?

3. How do you feel about illness, disability, aging, or other signs of physical mortality? Do you tend to avoid them, or can you confront them without shrinking?

4. What frightens you? Why?

5. What situations bring out your strengths and elicit your best functioning?

As you think about these questions, your heart may sink. You may wonder if you have the inner strength and the capability to cope with the demands that you are going to face.

Your fear and trepidation is a positive sign. It means you are a person who can let difficult ideas and uncomfortable feelings come into view so that they can be dealt with. Your concern is an indication that you can grow and become a more creative and better functioning person.

Helpers often say to themselves, "I can't handle this. I can't do this. Someone else would handle this much better." These same self-accusations are being made by the patient. For both patient and helpers, such self-criticism may serve as a way to avoid or delay facing up to reality. The "I can't" frame of mind is often an excuse to avoid the risk of failure.

In caring for chronic illness or disability there will be many occasions of failure and discouragement. They have to be expected and they have to be faced. To get to the renewal stage will require the ability to tolerate the inevitable mistakes.

Some of the tasks required of helpers are precise. The ambulance must be called. Medication must be taken. Arrangements must be made to care for the children. And so on.

These are the easiest tasks. It is much more difficult to handle the emotional pain of chronic illness. You cannot deal with the emotional pain the same way you can with precisely defined tasks. But there are ways to cope with it.

Listening is one of the most effective ways. That means real listening that attends to the patient's spoken and unspoken cries. Such listening is not easy. It arouses our fears for our own mortality, our frustration at being helpless in the face of unpredictable new realities. If you do not have the capability to listen to the emotional pain of the patient, do not hesitate to seek supportive counseling for yourself. One of the most important skills of the successful caregiver is this ability to listen in a way that helps the patient unload the tremendous burden of fear and pain that the illness or disability has aroused. The successful helper has the ability to regard the patient as someone worth listening to, someone to nurture in a continuing relationship.

A successful helper recognizes that it is not possible to make the illness or handicap disappear.

This point seems obvious. Yet it is the crux of a successful response to unavoidable change.

The patient does not have the choice of escaping the illness. There is no time off, no leaving the scene, no departing the sick room. A successful helper accepts this and faces the unavoidable changes squarely. It has happened and it is an inescapable part of the patient's life. But it is not the entirety of the patient, nor is it the only factor in the relationship between the patient and helper. A successful helper does the best that he can do, but realizes that perfection is never possible.

Helpers may be frustrated, disappointed, afraid—just as patients are. An honest, consistent, and realistic effort is what is required. Do your best and don't worry about achieving the unachievable.

Sometimes doing your best does not involve doing. Instead, it involves listening to the fear that is expressed in many different ways by the patient. It involves affirming that you will continue to be there to help face the fear.

There are things to be done. Often they are simple: opening or closing the curtains; reading aloud; talking quietly about subjects of mutual interest; asking for advice on matters about which the patient is especially knowledgeable. The patient may be too ill to seek out sources of gratifying mental stimulation so it is up to the helper to bring some form of stimulating activity or interchange into the patient's life.

The helper can take an active role in medical care for the patient. It may be necessary to provide help getting to and from the doctor's or therapist's office. Interpreting and remembering medical instructions is also often needed.

Help with getting dressed or undressed, bathing, combing, shaving, and other matters of personal grooming are quite important. The helper can scout ahead for restrooms that accommodate mobility devices.

Household bills, tax payments, and other financial and legal matters need to be addressed despite illness. Assistance is often needed in these areas. A person engaged in business will have ongoing business requirements that will not wait for a better time. This is another area where the trusted helper can assist with urgent needs.

In addition, household maintenance and repair does not abate during illness. The grass continues to grow, the snow falls on sidewalks, plumbing leaks occur, and so on and on. If there are children, their needs must still be attended to, and since the children will be under stress from their parent's illness, they may need extra encouragement to focus on their education and personal development.

Good helpers are invaluable for all of these matters. None of the customary, daily routine needs go away when illness strikes. The patient may be too ill, or too low in morale, to be able to organize and direct the work and the workforce needed to accomplish the tasks of daily family and business life. Family, friends, and other concerned helpers can provide this critically needed function.

Helpers, particularly members of the family, must take care of themselves, too. Just because a loved one is ill does not mean that your own responsibilities and needs will go away. You cannot abandon your own life. You must make good judgments about what it is possible for you to handle, and then act accordingly.

Do not make commitments you know you will be unable to keep. Don't take on tasks that make you so angry that you will add to the patient's problems. It is better to say no than to get embroiled in things that generate guilt, anger, and resentment for you. Your negative feelings will be all too clear to the patient. A simple, "No, I can't do that now because . . ." is better than trying to do it and being caught up in negative feelings.

Volunteer for what you know is reasonable for your own practical and emotional limitations. But know this: most people can do far more than they believe possible if they are drawing upon the love they feel for the patient. Most people can do far less than they believe when they allow anger and guilt and rage at fate to dominate their emotions. The positive emotion of love gives us strength and courage.

As a helper you will do well to recognize that there are a great many things that you cannot control. You cannot control the operating schedule in the hospital, or how many emergencies have thrown the doctor's schedule far behind. But as a helper you *can* influence some things. If there are delays in the medical schedule, you can ask if there is another doctor available, or if you can reschedule at a better time, or if a more comfortable place can be found for you and the patient to wait.

Do not be passive in today's medical setting!

There are a few things that you can actually control. Some of them may involve the patient. Most of them involve you.

You are the one who has control over your own response to frustration, delay, uncertainty, and other discouragements. You can control the development of alternative plans when the original plans go awry. You can also control your own willingness to seek out information, and to speak directly and factually to the people from whom you seek information or assistance.

Helpers need to learn to exercise control over their own perceptions, responses, and emotions so that they are effective in communicating, acting, and helping.

It is often the case that the patient wants something but does not ask. This can be frustrating. Perhaps he is unable to tell you. Perhaps he feels guilty about being sick, and about inconveniencing you. Whatever the reason, there is a problem for both patients and helpers when needs cannot be communicated. The helper can often deal with this by observing, "You seem uncomfortable." Then try offering a suggestion for amending the situation. "It looks like raising the bed might help." "Can I get the bedpan?", or whatever seems appropriate.

Whether or not the helper has hit on the right answer to the unstated need, the patient will often then be able to verbalize what is needed. It will be understood that your offer to help is genuine. That provides an emotional boost as well as the help that is needed.

If you don't get a positive reception to your suggestions, you might say, "None of these ideas seem useful to you right now." Try going on. "Would you like me to stay a little longer, or shall I look in later?"

If the response is "stay," then decide how long you are comfortable, or able, to stay—and say so. "Good. I don't have to leave for another 15 minutes."

If the response is "leave," then you can say, "Then we will plan on seeing each other . . ." and name a specific time for the next meeting.

The most difficult situation for the helper is when there is no response. Think of the stage that the patient may be in. There are some stages, as you have seen earlier, where the lack of response is not uncommon. Then think about the person. Do they retreat into silence when they are upset? If so, try taking their hand and saying nothing.

If anger is the likely cause of the silence, it may help to ask if they need some assistance in getting out from under the anger. Of course, you can't cure anger. But asking about it lets the patient know you are emotionally by their side and paying attention to them.

Some people are very verbal about anger. They may rage about their situation. Often enough, you may feel that you yourself are the target of the anger. You may feel misunderstood and hurt by the vehemence of the patient's anger. In this case, try something like this: "I hear you saying that all the rage and anger you feel right now was caused by something I said or did. If I understand the situation, you started to get upset when you were told the results of your tests (or whatever the cause of the upset may have been). Are there questions we need to ask the doctor? Are there things we need to do? I am sorry you feel so much fear and anger now." When you have a good relationship you can add, "I am not leaving. Even though this is an upsetting situation for both of us, you can count on me."

Sometimes, these words do not help. This is often because the past relationship has created a context in which it is difficult to work through anger and accusations. In such a case, offer the hope that you will be able to work things out. It may be desirable to offer the idea that a third party (a professional, not a friend) can help set things right.

Conclude by saying, "I am willing to keep trying. What about you?" Often direct, simple, non-punitive confrontation is desirable.

Some patients have a history of verbal explosiveness where destructive words flow too freely. Confront this with words such as, "This kind of anger is not good for either one of us. I will come back when you are calmer and we can talk about it more rationally."

Illness may provide the opportunity to change unproductive and harmful ways of being together. This is because illness puts the unproductive patterns into stark focus. The crisis of illness may lead to a crisis of relationships. But crisis is an opportunity for emotional restructuring and healing. This can occur when the motivation is to preserve and enhance the relationship.

Helpers, like patients, look for guarantees. If such and such a plan of treatment is followed then everything will turn out all right. Chronic illness and disability are conditions with no guarantees. You must be content with knowing only what the next step is that you are going to try.

With any unavoidable change, as with life in general, we can only know what has happened and what is happening now. We can make decisions about the next steps to take. Perhaps we can estimate the odds that the next step will lead in the direction we hope to go. But there is always uncertainty about the future.

Unavoidable change produces loss and anxiety. It also produces curiosity about the future, which we cannot predict. For those who are comfortable with risks and with the unknown, the changes may bring excitement, an opportunity for reprioritizing goals, and an opportunity to reaffirm strongly held inner values.

It is important to respond to unavoidable changes by using the changes to deepen the meaningfulness of each day. Do not respond inappropriately. An example of this would be the decision to buy a new wardrobe, or to go off on a fling, or take some other uncharacteristic and foolish action because life has been drastically altered by unavoidable changes. Such responses usually end up having highly negative consequences. They create guilt and shame. They threaten relationships. They reinforce the anxiety and fear that the responses may have temporarily submerged. Unpleasant external realities are best faced by strong internal responses to the fear and anger that have been created.

When someone you care about is going through an unavoidable life change, focus your efforts on the things you can directly affect and control—your own feelings, attitudes, and desire to help the person you care for. Improve your inner strength by facing the facts as they are. Do not try to avoid the facts, either for yourself or for the patient. When the patient says, "I am in pain," it is not helpful to you, or the patient, to say they are imagining it, or it can't be so bad. Neither denial nor reassurances may be the best approach. It is usually more important to listen, hear, and recognize the reality of the patient's condition.

Finally, illness and disability are grim and difficult. But that does not mean that the capacity for pleasure, joy, satisfaction, diversion, interest in other people, love of nature, intellectual curiosity, and sensual stimulation have been lost.

Being ill or handicapped limits the range of responses. It limits the emotional and physical energy that is available. But it does not change the bedrock nature of the individual.

All of us are people with passions, and illness or disability does not change our passionate nature. Being treated as a person with passions is very healing. It is far different from being treated as a person who is a shell or a shadow from whom all human passions have been removed. Illness or disability may change the focus of our passion or the response to it. It does not, however, change the need for passion in emotional engagements.

Now it is time to turn more directly to the needs of the helpers themselves. Under the stress of uncertainty caused by illness and disability, helpers may fail to notice their own symptoms of distress. Some of these symptoms absolutely require outside intervention. In other cases, helpers may focus almost exclusively on their own symptoms of distress, and become completely preoccupied. This, too, may require outside intervention.

Listed below are a number of clues to your own possible distress. If any of them persist, you need to contact your family physician or mental health counselor. You are suffering, and you deserve professional care.

1. Inability to sleep or to eat enough to meet minimum health requirements. (For these symptoms, three or four days warrant a call for professional help.)

2. Feeling that it is impossible to get rested or nourished, no matter how much one sleeps or eats.

3. Feelings of dread or panic anytime the phone rings, whenever it is necessary to face the patient, when there are meetings with medical personnel, or even just when it involves normal contacts.

4. The use of alcohol or drugs to relax, forget, or feel good.

5. Any changes in the quantity of prescribed medications you take.

6. Any use whatsoever of the medication prescribed for the patient. (This is very serious and requires immediate attention.)

7. A sense of guilt that takes the form of not being able to face the patient or even the mundane tasks of the day.

8. Inability to think about anything other than the medical problems that you and the patient face.

9. Any behavior that is out of character, such as changes in spending habits, manner of dress, personal hygiene, irritability, and so forth.

10. The growth of fantasy and increasing avoidance of reality and responsibility.

Any of these is an indication that the ability to function effectively is impaired.

They are not signs of moral decay or character failure. Helpers facing the difficult challenges of illness and disability often succumb to pressures that they cannot handle alone.

If these symptoms persist they can lead to the impairment of judgment. They are signs of anxiety and depression. Physical symptoms of stress can also occur. These physical, emotional, and psychological conditions can be treated. Sometimes they are treated medically, sometimes by counseling alone. Sometimes, both methods are useful. You owe it to yourself and to the patient you care for to deal with stress-related symptoms. They can all too easily impair your life, and the life of the patient.

There are times when a helper has done all that is humanly possible to do on behalf of the ill person. Then, trying to do more is not helpful. Not only is it not helpful, the quality of your life will be severely damaged. In such cases, you need to get more help from others. In fact, in most cases of helper burnout the helper has been unwilling or unable to ask for assistance from others.

Just as we have talked about the need for patients to learn to ask for help, helpers also must learn to ask for help.

The appendix to this book contains a list of agencies and organizations that provide support and services for chronic illness and disability. They can be very useful for helpers. This list is in addition to your own family, friends, and the various professionals available within the community. Ask for help before you sacrifice yourself.

Helping a chronically ill or disabled person can be an exhausting, difficult, and stressful task. The above paragraphs have emphasized the negative consequences that helpers can suffer.

If that was all there was to it helping would not be something that many people would undertake. But there is another side to helping.

Helping others is a personally rewarding, satisfying, enriching experience. For every moment of fear, anger, exhaustion, or concern, there can be a moment of joy, pleasure, and satisfaction.

At the end, the relationships we build and nurture with other human beings are the most important triumphs of life. There are no more rewarding or uplifting relationships than those that are developed between helpers and the person that they help.

CHAPTER EIGHT

CONCLUSION

You probably recognized yourself in the stages that have been presented in this book. Almost everyone experiences the emotional responses that have been described.

Let's review the major characteristics of each stage. What can we, as patients, expect to feel? How can we respond to the powerful emotions unleashed by illness?

Illness is emotionally and physically depriving. It is also frightening, for it thrusts great uncertainties into our lives. At each stage, our responses to the fear and deprivation are different.

As patients, we forever let go of the idea that life is going to be easy. Instead we look for ways to savor the life that is ours. This is a tall order, for life is now hard, worrisome, and may even seem intolerable. But we must learn to get through life by using our abilities as adaptive human beings to be flexible. We must become committed to the value of small joys and small successes. We must resolve the problems that now face us with flexibility and an openness to alternate ways of living. Emotional well-being can be built on what we can do and on what we can enjoy. It can never be built on thinking about what cannot be done and what can no longer be enjoyed.

As we review each stage, look inside yourself. See what helpful understanding you would offer to another at each point. Then, offer yourself that same understanding and support.

CRISIS

During the stage I call crisis, the patient is beset by a major physical illness. The patient is too ill to be responsible for anything but the next breath, and even that may require the help of a respirator. All emotional and physical energy is directed toward survival and the beginning of healing.

The patient is often too sick even to be frightened. Events are often confused. Time is distorted and may pass unnoticed. Disorientation, a feeling of being lost, is common.

At these times, we fall back on our innate biological ability to heal. If the crisis is one of many in a short time, a good portion of our resilience is exhausted. With low reserves, there need to be others who will bring energy and adaptability. Family, friends, medical personnel, even strangers can help.

By and large, everyone responds well in a crisis. Family and friends are usually unflagging in their efforts to make sure that the patient is being cared for properly. Others may assist with the patient's financial responsibilities; friends may provide food, child care, and home maintenance; the patient's medical care is in the hands of others.

Everyone knows the patient is terribly ill. And they respond. Unfortunately, those most affected by the patient's illness do not always receive the support and help they need at this time. Family and friends are often exhausted by the demands the situation places upon them. The children of a very ill parent are often neglected in the concern for the patient. Help is needed for them. Often, a show of concern and active support and assistance are very welcome.

At the worst, family members desert the ill person, or they compete with the ill person for attention. This happens because such persons are overwhelmed. They do not have enough emotional sturdiness. At a later time, the patient will need to find ways to release the bitterness caused by feeling abandoned. At the best, the patient is not abandoned and gets the needed attention. Those helping the patient are able to ask for and to get relief from the arduous duties of patient care and family responsibilities. There will be outlets for enjoyment and relaxation—relaxing with a book or music or a movie or favorite TV program, or playing with children or pets. Each person will find relief in something different. Such diversion is essential at this stage. (However, the abuse of alcohol or drugs to escape anxiety can only complicate the situation for everyone concerned.) A period of crisis is not a death watch to be marked by the shunning of all pleasurable activities. A period of crisis is a life watch. The patient needs a hand to hold. And the person extending the hand to the patient needs someone's shoulder to lean on.

ISOLATION

The isolation stage is insidious. It occurs just as the patient is coming to the full realization that the condition will not go away. There will be no full recovery. There will always be the fear of another recurrence.

The family, friends, or other helpers who have devoted themselves to "doing" (by engaging in intense activity) to escape from anxiety are now fatigued emotionally. Without making a conscious choice, patients and helpers withdraw into themselves. In other words, they isolate themselves from one another. They do not want to burden others with their fears. Perhaps the idea that they are afraid is kept secret. This is especially true for those who go through marked episodes of the isolation phase.

In Chapter Two, Evie's husband was a man of action and he was uncomfortable expressing his feelings in words. "Doing" for Evie was his best, and only way, to express his love for her. Evie was even less able to talk about her feelings. Since her illness her normal ways of "doing" for her husband were not possible. Evie and her husband provide us with an example of the emotional pain experienced during the isolation phase. Patients often do not experience themselves as vibrant contributors in the world. This is particularly problematic since contacts with others are important, lending a sense of perspective and reinforcing the feeling that one is worthy, even though beseiged by circumstances.

The patient's anxiety often produces a stiffness, in dealings with others or with oneself. There is a belief, usually partially justified, that no one can understand the devastation caused by physical decline—the losses or changes in one's abilities and self-image. Isolation most troubles independent patients (people whose past lifestyle has been one of "I can do it all alone").

Indeed, much can still be done alone. But what can be done is not in the realm of activity the patient has learned to credit yet. Family, friends, and helpers can aid by acknowledging the intense upset caused by the life changes forced by illness, while being actively supportive of the patient's struggle to hang on to as much independence as possible.

Friends, family, and helpers often feel unappreciated when, worn out from the crisis stage, they discover the patient does not credit their contributions. Everyone needs acknowledgement. But helpers need to remember that the patient is probably not aware of what has been provided. There is no need to browbeat the patient with these facts. The mutual respect and desire to help one another that is characteristic of well-functioning families should prevail. As soon as anyone adopts a martyr's stance—"look what I have given up for you"—the results are sure to be damaging. It is a fact of life that no matter how much we do for ourselves or others, we will not receive all the affirmation we desire.

The first rule in breaking the isolation is that open communications are vital. Blame must play no part. "We've all had a rough time" is a very different remark from "No one cares how hard it has been for me." Talking about feelings is very important.

"I've been caught up in the sadness of my physical situation. I'm afraid I have not been listening to you." Such a statement works to reestablish (or even establish for the first time) a sense of caring and of togetherness. It is necessary to lighten up the emotional load by communication and sharing. It is necessary to find ways to break the isolation.

ANGER

Chronic illness does not disappear. Nor are there any quick fixes to the damage to self-esteem. Anger is the usual response to the interruption of life by illness. Everyone involved becomes more consciously angry. But angry at what?

Again, patient and helpers may see things differently. And both distort reality. The reality is straightforward. A cataclysmic change in one's image of oneself, or of one's partner or friend, has occurred. It is natural to be terrified, and it is profoundly comforting to have an enemy to blame.

But the anguish is often focused inappropriately. Such beliefs as "You brought this on yourself," or "Look what a lemon I got stuck with" are fear responses. The fear invades all who recognize that they too will crumble physically at some point.

Patients frequently ascribe evil to themselves. "I must have done something terrible to deserve this." Most patients turn the anger inward and become their own judge, jury, and prosecutor. We can understand this by recognizing how frightening mortality is for most people. Patients feel a loss of control over their lives. "I don't deserve this, and want to get out," is a strong feeling. Wanting to escape has everything to do with recognizing the cruel reality while continuing to believe that you are entitled to normal human passions and impulses.

There may be no way to satisfy some of the basic needs for independence, safety, or sexuality. But there is always a way to break such basic needs into smaller objectives. Attaining these can provide satisfaction.

The patient can make many decisions about things to be done for or to him. It is important that this much independence and autonomy be respected. Treating the patient as an incompetent can only heat the flames of anger.

There are times when it seems that everyone is angry. A devoted and hardworking spouse may begin to feel overwhelmed, then resentful. Impatience will be clearly communicated to the ill loved one. In such a situation, direct action is necessary.

I have seen many cases where the patient has spent much energy applauding the behavior of a spouse or other helper. In every such case, there also exists a deep resentment because the patient feels that the spouse or helper is complaining—and complaining about things the patient would give several eye teeth to be able to do.

In these circumstances, a quiet, non-angry talk about how one feels is mandatory. These conversations are a necessary beginning to clarify one's emotional needs. When both sides participate, each has the satisfaction of contributing to the well-being of the other.

Patients often feel unworthy of the care they have received. This sense of unworthiness is easily converted to resentment and anger. It can lead to a feeling that everyone else is angry, too. In truth, each person *is* angry—but at an uncaring fate.

If the anger becomes too strong, patients should yell at the broom or tear up old newspapers. Fear and anger are disruptive emotions engendered by a sense of loss of control. Patients need to begin to regain control. However, they must take back that control in small steps. If patients bite off too large a task, they set themselves up for certain failure and more anger.

The hardest task of all is to notice what can still be appreciated. The ill spouse may still be the only person who can listen intelligently to an account of the day. The well spouse may be the only one who knows what kind of book can provide respite from physical and emotional torment.

The basic reasons for the anger, in most cases, cannot be avoided. And, it does no good to assign blame. The response must be to become task-oriented. "Today I will walk the length of my room when I get upset, or call a friend, or answer one inquiry."

Everyone involved must stick to reality, to what is possible. A little housecleaning can be emotionally cleansing. Doing hand laundry is a task with a short term, satisfying conclusion. These are the kinds of tasks that add greatly to the feeling of being in control. In later stages, patients will be able to modify their overly rigid needs for control.

Patients must use their strengths to do what they can do. Striving toward a goal, even in small doses, is an antidote to anger. If patients cannot remember what strengths remain, they should be reminded. Patients, family, friends, and helpers should all focus on the strengths that remain, on the accomplishments that can still be achieved. This basic rule is a key to dealing with anger. There also needs to be a recognition that anger causes feelings of pain that can't be wished away.

RECONSTRUCTION

At some point the process of reconstruction begins. It comes sooner to those who credit themselves with strengths. Reconstruction is helped along if the illness has subsided enough that more energy is available.

Reconstruction does not mean a physical cure. What it does mean is that the patient has discovered some ways to be effective despite physical limitations. Fighting to open the food package can be frustrating and defeating. But if one can contain the agitation long enough to thoroughly examine the mechanism, and to ask for help with what cannot be done personally, a very important accomplishment has been achieved that signals reconstruction.

I remember my real pleasure when, after my visual impairment, I was able to avoid running into walls. This sounds like a very simple skill for an educated adult, but I found it very hard to do. I became quite gleeful when I could sense and avoid hazards in my own house. Then, with the aid of a seeing-eye cat whose affection was unshakable, and a growing, competent daughter who warned of hazards as I lost the ability to detect them, life felt momentarily as if it were moving along.

I want to stress the fleeting nature of these good feelings. Often people do well for a few weeks and then are devastated by an incident that is significant to them alone. But each experience that involves trusting and succeeding is a building block for the next step. When the calmer, more focused feelings leave us, there can be room for confidence that they will return another day. Each day is its own story. Often, each hour of the day acquaints us more deeply with all of the emotional stages.

INTERMITTENT DEPRESSION

As the patient becomes more comfortable with limitations, family and friends may lapse into an "everything is fine" stance. Everything may be a whole lot better, but there is no guarantee for the future. The rug is apt to be pulled out from under one's feet repeatedly.

Should this happen, expect feelings of depression, helplessness, and hopelessness. After all, everything possible was done to prevent such an eventuality—and still it occurred.

These feelings are real and reactive to each new turn in the illness. The feelings of depression, helplessness, and hopelessness can also arise from an increasing concern about the illness. Just as one does not berate friends who suffer from circumstances beyond their control or their ability to anticipate, one must not berate one's self for changes in their illness. Patients must believe that at some level, no matter how deep or disguised, they matter. This belief must then be translated into action.

I have patients who reassure themselves, when necessary, that things could be worse: Maybe they have one good friend, or maybe they can still enjoy hot fudge sundaes, or maybe they can follow a difficult medical regime meticulously, or maybe they can listen to another person's self-doubts without trying to compete.

Depression is heightened by a lack of stimulation. Finding something that will make the juices flow is very helpful in keeping depression at bay. Some patients search for the most obnoxious disc jockey in their area and then notice their responses to him. No one can take these responses away. They are valid. Feeling them helps to ease the grip of depression.

We all have periods when we feel overmatched and not up to the struggle. But as long as we pay attention to the struggle, we will get through the day. We flounder when we set unrealistic standards, or cannot grieve for what has been lost, or cannot start each day afresh.

Depression can be tackled despite the morass of physical complications that tries to drag us down.

RENEWAL

Those who have intervals of renewal are not simply lucky. They are indeed fortunate, but the good fortune is won with great effort—the continuing effort of making each day as much as it can be. Interludes of renewal are delicate treasures; like a lovely balloon, they may float away or burst. But they can be still created anew.

The creation of renewal comes from the experiences that teach us not to waste the present on fearing the future. We are capable of more risk-taking than we believe possible, and often this power comes to the fore when we become ill. It is an arduous task to accept oneself, one's life, and to accept others. Yet we learn to credit those things we like in ourselves, and to be tolerant toward all that we dislike. (These likes and dislikes go far beyond what has happened to us physically.) The credit and the tolerance are what build emotional strength.

I would not have believed any of this 15 years ago. It would have sounded too easy. My patients at that time were suffering deeply. I was not optimistic about being able to guide them toward the flexible use of options in their lives. I could perceive these options, but they could not. I learned how important it is to have someone who can help you focus your attention in the most productive way.

When you are sick, you may have trouble transferring all the positive skills of a lifetime to coping with illness, limitation, frustration, and sorrow. The daily effort of making each day more than a grinding endurance test may seem overwhelming, but life *can* be more than endurance. How much more will depend, in part, on your experience coping with or overcoming physical limitations before the onset of your illness. If you have trained as an athlete, for example, you will be more familiar with pushing your body beyond your expected limitations.

You have seen from earlier chapters that I do not minimize the severity of the problems chronic illness introduces. Those who minimize miss the whole point. From a psychological perspective, the question is what happens when your options are limited, and what coping skills can you use to identify and maximize your available options. The positive coping skills explored in this book and summarized below are the same ones necessary to cope with any situation involving marked frustration and loss—unavoidable health changes require these skills.

Make Your Expectations Realistic

Whenever I urge you to have realistic expectations, I know some of you will have a sinking feeling. One of the problems with illness is that you may feel one way when you get up in the morning and quite a different way an hour later. So, how do you recognize what is realistic? How do you make plans? How do you predict?

The most important aspect of making expectations realistic is the recognition that they are time-limited. Try to ask yourself, "What can I do on the basis of how I feel right now?"

Health changes such as chronic physical illness throw so many obstacles in the way of the use of time that they can rob you of your entire sense of predictable time. What do we do when we have available time and we feel a certain way? What kind of expectations do we want to make for ourselves to be sure we will make good use of that time? Obviously, a great deal of time goes into the management of the illness itself, but beyond that, there is a host of things that need to be accomplished. Initially, the list of things to do gets longer and more confusing as you add the "want to's" to the "have to's." The bottom line is: if you have two minutes, what are you going to do with them? I counsel people to check with themselves to find out what they want to do. It is important for you to do this because illness can make you feel that you must surrender all of your goals, all of your wishes.

From your list of "want to's," check inside to see what you have the emotional energy for. Make your expectations work like this: Within the limits of my physical ability I will do whatever it is I want to do, for however long I can do it. Expectations need to be time limited. You do not tell yourself, I am going to graduate from law school in three years. It is really a question of what you can do right now without harming yourself. For all goal-directed people, who have been able to count on themselves to achieve a certain level of productivity in a certain length of time, this particular skill is very, very difficult to learn. On the surface, it feels like it goes counter to everything they have been doing. It does not. You are just trying to make the time you have count. However, you may get in your own way by criticizing yourself for what you cannot do, rather than focusing on what you can do. Your focus on what you can do must be able to change with the ebb and flow of your energy level.

Approach Problems Actively

A second skill, following closely behind realistic expectations, is taking an active approach to problems. There is so much forced passivity that comes with illness that you may begin to feel you are also a psychologically inactive person. This feeling causes, and is the essence of, depression. And depression can be more limiting than the chronic illness itself.

What is an active approach? It consists of defining the problem, and then determining what outcome you want from the effort you spend on solving it. It involves trying to ensure that any energy you expend constitutes a step toward a solution. Rarely does it constitute the complete solution. You will probably have to muffle the impulse to assume responsibility for the total task. "I cannot" is at times the most active way to promote and protect yourself. The admission "I cannot do something" is often the first step to solving a problem realistically.

What you can do is define what it is you want, and then use every ounce of creativity you possess to determine how you are going to make it happen. Creativity is *not* impaired by chronic illness. Suppose, for example, you had always done a lot of entertaining in your pre-illness days and now you want to increase your social contacts. The first step is to acknowledge that you cannot entertain in the same fashion as you have previously. Then you need to determine who you wish to see and set up a meeting place and time, subject to change depending on how you feel. There are some high emotional hurdles in this scenario: letting go of your past self-image, deciding who you are currently comfortable with, and, hardest of all, making a date with the understanding that it may need to be postponed.

After you define the problem, you need to figure out how many facets there are to achieving some kind of resolution to it. The next step is to then expect yourself to complete only that part of the effort that is realistic. What this means is that you need a broader sense of community than might have been necessary in your pre-illness days. There are going to be any number of things you cannot do alone, but your dreams do not all have to change. But how they are realized will probably change. It is absolutely essential that you hang on to what you want, what you hope for, and what engages your passions. Your mission is to get as much satisfaction as possible using your energies in creative and flexible ways.

If, as your physical limitations decrease, you are able to increase your emotional abilities, your chances for experiencing satisfaction are heightened. For those of you who are newly diagnosed, this may not make a lot of sense yet. You have not had the time to incorporate the experience and perspective of this new-found emotional awareness since the onset of your illness. The trauma and its grief may still be too fresh. You may still be listening to an internal, critical voice that says: "I cannot and that is bad" rather than "I cannot, so how can I get it done?" Illness initially forces you into passivity. Your responses are limited, sometimes frozen by fear. But as you learn to quiet your internal critic, you will have increased energy for other people in your world. And seeing yourself as part of a social matrix opens you up for compassion, trust, and hope.

Seek Appropriate Help

The next skill is to learn to ask for appropriate help. When you are very sick and frightened, you need a different kind of help than you do on an easier day. You can expect to encounter a variety of internal resistances at different times to either asking for help or relinquishing it. Even so, this is an area where almost everyone I have met has eventually been able to grow. Asking for help can become a more graceful skill.

It is not a moral weakness to ask for assistance, though many of you may regard asking for help as shameful. But, it is a major limitation if you do not know how to determine whether or not assistance is appropriate. (It is also a limitation if you are harsh and angry with your helper.) If you are fortunate in being an accurate self-observer, or in having someone who can tell you when you are not being constructive, much can be done with this coping skill. Asking for help is certainly not the first choice for people who would rather do everything themselves, but it should be your choice if you are going to pursue what you need and want when you cannot do it alone. Having what you need and want leads to a much happier life than does the bitterness that comes from feeling that everything has been impaired by having to ask for help.

If you have a very hard time asking for help, there is an easy way to learn how to do this: Consider what you would do if you were fully able-bodied and a friend of yours had your particular problem to solve. What would you do? Do you see yourself denying help as you fear others might deny you? Would you be perturbed if your friend asked for the specific help that was required? Chances are you would feel fine about helping out if you could. You would just do it in the course of events—no problem. Try to be as kind to yourself as you would be to another.

Handle Your Anger

The next skill involves learning how to become emotionally efficient and energy conscious. Energy is a tremendous problem for those with chronic illnesses—there is none to waste. Any energy that is expended in a way that is not nourishing is a waste. Some of the most wasteful expenditures are brought on by resentment and anger. These emotions are not bad, but they do wear you out.

If you are angry, it helps to have some consciousness of what you are angry about, and whether you want to be angry about it. Sometimes you want to be angry because that's the appropriate and effective response. Sometimes you will want to be angry because it is more efficient to be openly angry than to deal with bitterness or other forms of calcified anger. The better you get at being direct about anger early on, the more energy you will save, and the more efficient you will be. You can say to yourself, "Aha! I'm irritated." Surprisingly, many people do not know how to recognize their own irritation. If you are feeling irritated, it might be helpful to be assertive, even if in the short run you feel uncomfortable.

What all these coping skills have in common is that they are daily necessities. You don't just get it down pat once and then forget about it—you need to use these skills frequently. Every day is going to give you something different to try to manage.

Participate

Another skill which helps with any loss, but is especially restorative for those with chronic illness, is to put positive energy back into the world. You can do this with your family, friends, with self-help groups connected with your illness, or with community groups. Put your talents, your compassion, your knowledge, and your experience out there in a way that will benefit others. To fully participate, you must be a good friend to yourself, fully valuing your finer qualities.

If asking for help is a skill you already possess, then you possess more constructive energy to invest in the world around you. Obviously, one of the things illness can do is to constrict your social world. Sometimes this leads to a perception that there is nothing you can do for others. That is just flat-out wrong. If you have exhausted your own creativity, flexibility, and that of your friends in looking for a way to participate in the world around you, call such organizations as the Arthritis Foundation and other research or self-help organizations for suggestions. (See the Appendix for a listing.) People don't volunteer because there is nothing else to do; they do it because it feels good.

For those of us with children, there is a constant access route to return positive energy to the environment. If we are sensitive to the self-esteem needs of our children by being positive and supportive, that positive support will be reciprocated.

Live in the Present

Another skill that is a challenge to learn, due to the traumatic nature of illness, is to look neither too far backward nor too far forward. With illness comes the loss of the sense of invulnerability—that we have a protective bubble around us—that nothing bad can happen. Of course, bad things can happen and they did when you became ill. But if you are only looking backward, you are giving up on yourself emotionally all the time. True, your losses are major issues, but losses do not get people through one day at a time, or one day after another. Losses are not a good reason for living, and they do not provide a way to have fun. If you use all your emotional energy considering how things were before the illness, and compare it to how things are now, you end up punishing yourself. All you will see is how badly off you are right now. If you sense this going on, you need to be extremely aggressive about rejecting this attitude.

Illness does not diminish one's humanity! It just does not. Mobility and physical comfort decrease with illness.

Fear and worry increase. But illness does not diminish your humanity. Be kind to yourself. Avoid dwelling on how good things were compared to how they are now. Also, try to avoid distant-future fantasies. There is no way to know on the basis of today what will be there years hence. And, you know, there never has been a way to know how things will be in the future. Try to keep yourself grounded where you are. If you are not stuck in the past, or tormented by distant-future images of what should be, you will have the opportunity to manage each day with awareness. Living in the moment with consciousness, patience, compassion, and appreciation of yourself, and others, lets you get on with life in a creative fashion, in spite of the pain of your losses.

Cherish the Good Times

The last skill I would recommend to you is to pay attention to the positives. This can only be done if you have already mastered the skill of living fully in the moment. If you go through every 24 hours with enough of yourself available to the world, when something positive happens, you will let it in. There were rainbows yesterday, but there have not been rainbows in a while. However, there may be an interesting interaction between you and the grocery clerk, or the paper boy might get the paper on the porch so you won't begin your day frustrated, or you have a close, warm exchange with someone you care about. These are the kinds of positive moments I mean.

These are moments that can be framed. They are complete and need to be stored and used on days when life is much harder. If we put ourselves in an open frame of mind, we increase the likelihood of noticing the positives that are already there. If we are in a quagmire of negative emotion and perception, we can turn anything into proof that there are only painful things in the world.

The final skill is learning to hold onto these positives. To cherish them sufficiently so that they do not drop out of your repertoire of significant life events. Once you are able to notice the positives, how do you hold onto them? The best way is to slow down—to use relaxation, meditation, and your own internal capacity for joy to feel that given moment inside. Let it resonate within. This allows your emotional commitment to be fully focused on the process of life. Part of your goal is to be as emotionally able-hearted as possible, despite your physical limitations.

For me, this is still a daily issue. I am able to do work that I like. In this I am fortunate. My daughter's ever-increasing independence and emotional growth also help me keep an outward focus.

When my daughter was little it was painful not to be able to see her as she trotted off to visit a friend. But it was a pleasure to watch her as an indistinct whirling dervish in a classroom play. How much nicer that I could get an enormous enlargement of her twinkling form from a photo taken by a friend. These days, classroom drama has given way to adolescent competence. What my disabilities mean to her continues to change, and there is still important work for both of us to do.

When she was small, Jacynth used to say, "You are the only Mama I have." This was a chastisement as much as it was a compliment. Our struggle with my disabilities is part of the ongoing expansion of our relationship. She learns from me that there can be both joy and sorrow in life. She learns that we can face life either way.

Years ago, when my only significant disability was partial blindness, I picked Jacynth up, carried her a short way, then missed a step. Down we went like Humpty Dumpty. Jacynth cried from surprise, but one of her little friends came up and said, "My Mama could never do that. That was neat." How we see things is so important. The child's perception of what happened recast my emotional response to the event. I have tried to keep paramount this idea of how to see things.

At times, the circumstances you face may be miserable. Nothing can alter this reality. But you as a person do not need to be redeemed from circumstances. Trust that you will learn from each stage and from each cycle through the stages. Learn to trust others enough so that when the situation seems unbearably stressful, outside counseling and psychotherapy can be sought. Renewal cannot always be attained without help.

If this book has reached out to you at any level, you have already begun the process of renewal. You are adapting in the face of great difficulty. There is no right way to come through the ravages of unavoidable health changes. But I have tried to show you ways to remain an active agent in your own life. No matter how fatigued you become, use the awareness of your ability to actively affect your own life. Use your strong feelings to gain power and vitality.

You are not alone. None of us is alone. We may not know each other yet, but we are kindred spirits. A single treasured personal relationship makes the path bearable.

Each time you read this book, it will mean more to you. You will see yourself in new ways—ways that will yield a host of satisfactions.

I wish you a safe and thoughtful journey on what truly is a road of hope. I travel it with you. You have a companion, and you have hope.

APPENDIX

Listed below are some of the organizations that provide information and support to families and patients who have to cope with chronic pain or illness. Most of these organizations have local branches. To find out the location or contact person for your local group, get in touch with the national offices listed below.

In many areas, you will find support groups that do not have an affiliation with a national organization. You may learn about these from your physician, church, friends, neighbors, social service agencies, or in the community listings section of your local newspaper or telephone directory. (If you wish to suggest an organization for inclusion in our next edition, please contact the publisher.)

The first list begins with organizations whose primary focus is chronic pain. The others are grouped alphabetically by illness.

NATIONAL SELF-HELP CLEARINGHOUSE

25 West 43rd Street
Room 620
New York, NY 10036
212-642-2944

The clearinghouse began in 1976 to provide referral services, training, speakers, library, and other helpful information. It is a non-membership organization.

NATIONAL CHRONIC PAIN OUTREACH ASSOCIATION

7979 Old Georgetown Road
Suite 100
Bethesda, MD 20814-2429
301-652-4948

The association, founded in 1976, disseminates information and assists in the formation of local support groups. It has audiotapes and a variety of publications, including the quarterly *Lifeline*. There is a membership fee.

AIDS

NATIONAL ASSOCIATION OF PEOPLE WITH AIDS

1413 K Street NW
7th Floor
Washington, D.C. 20005
202-898-0414

This is the primary national organization for local AIDS support groups. Founded in 1987, it trains and assists over 100 community-based organizations. It offers a wide range of programs. There is a membership fee.

ALLERGIES & RESPIRATORY AILMENTS

AMERICAN LUNG ASSOCIATION

1740 Broadway
New York, NY 10019
212-315-8700
800-586-4872

This large organization was founded in 1904 and now has 59 state groups. It has a very broad focus that encompasses both patients and professionals. They produce a variety of informational publications.

ASTHMA & ALLERGY FOUNDATION OF AMERICA

1125 15th Street NW, Suite 502
Washington, D.C. 20005
202-466-7643
800-727-8462

Directed at both the public and professionals, the foundation is devoted to solving health problems posed by allergic diseases. They sponsor research and training, provides information, education, and library, and a speakers bureau. Twenty-five local branches have formed since its founding in 1953. They publish a newsletter.

NATIONAL ALLERGY & ASTHMA NETWORK

3554 Chain Bridge Road
Suite 200
Fairfax, VA 22030-2709
703-385-4403
800-878-4403

Founded in 1985, the network helps parents deal with the practical aspects of raising asthmatic children. *MA Report* is their monthly publication.

NATIONAL FOUNDATION FOR THE CHEMICALLY HYPERSENSITIVE

1158 North Huron Road
Lynwood, MI 48634
517-697-3989

Since its inception in 1986, the foundation has established 40 regional groups. Its focus is on both patients and professionals, including information, networking, data gathering, research, referrals, speakers bureaus, and a library. It publishes the quarterly *Cheers*. There is a membership fee.

AMPUTATION

AMERICAN AMPUTEE FOUNDATION

Box 250218, Hillcrest Station
Little Rock, AR 72225
501-666-2523

Founded in 1975, the foundation provides peer counseling, legal assistance, information, referrals, and rehabilitation. It also publishes the biennial *National Resource Directory*.

AMPUTEES IN MOTION

PO Box 2703
Escondido, CA 92033
619-454-9300

This is an organization formed to help amputees and their families reestablish an active life. A newsletter is published three times a year. There is a membership fee.

NATIONAL AMPUTATION FOUNDATION

73 Church Street
Malverne, NY 11565
516-887-3600

Founded in 1919, the foundation currently serves veterans and civilians alike. It helps with employment and social and mental rehabilitation. It also maintains a library and publishes *The Amp* newsletter monthly.

ALS

AMYOTROPHIC LATERAL SCLEROSIS ASSOCIATION

21021 Ventura Boulevard, Suite 321
Woodland Hills, CA 91364
818-340-7500
800-782-4747

Founded in 1985, the association has over 250,000 members in 135 regional groups.

ARTHRITIS

NATIONAL ARTHRITIS & MUSCULOSKELETAL & SKIN DISEASES INFORMATION CLEARINGHOUSE

One AMS Circle
Bethesda, MD 20892-3675
301-495-4484

The clearinghouse collects, publishes, and disseminates information for both patients and professionals.

ARTHRITIS FOUNDATION

1314 Spring Street Northwest
Atlanta, GA 30309
404-872-7100
800-283-7800

Founded in 1948, the foundation has 71 local groups with 700,000 members. The American Juvenile Arthritis Organization comes under its umbrella as well. It has several publications, including the bimonthly *Arthritis Today*. There is a membership fee.

CANCER

AMERICAN CANCER SOCIETY

1599 Clifton Road Northeast
Atlanta, GA 30329
404-320-3333
800-227-2345

The society was founded in 1913 and is an enormous organization with both regional and local branches. It sponsors many subgroups focused on specific populations, such as women with breast cancer. It also publishes a wide variety of publications for professionals and the public.

ROSE KUSHNER BREAST CANCER ADVISORY CENTER

PO Box 224
Kensington, MD 20895
301-897-3445

The center is a service group for people with breast cancer. Founded in 1975, it offers referrals and distributes Rose Kushner's book *If You've Thought about Breast Cancer*.

CANCER CARE

1180 Avenue of the Americas
New York, NY 10036
212-221-3300

Founded in 1944, this organization promotes and aids the development of social services for cancer patients and their families. It offers counseling and limited financial assistance, as well as supporting research and advocacy. Its publications include a newsletter.

CANCER CARING CENTER

4117 Liberty Avenue
Pittsburgh, PA 15224
412-622-1212

Founded in 1988, the center helps patients cope with the psychological impact of their disease. Services include self-help groups, a lending library, professional counseling, and a telephone help line. They also publish a newsletter. All services are free.

CANCER INFORMATION SERVICE

31 Center Drive
MSC2580 Building 31
Room 10A07
Bethesda, MD 20892-2580
800-422-6237

Founded in 1975 by the National Cancer Institute, the trained counselors provide information on the causes and prevention of cancer, as well as treatment and clinical trials for cancer patients.

CANDLELIGHTERS CHILDHOOD CANCER FOUNDATION

7910 Woodmont Avenue
Suite 460
Bethesda, MD 20814
301-657-8404
800-366-2223

This broad based international organization was founded in 1970 for parents of children with cancer. It offers guidance and emotional support, serves as a clearinghouse and liaison, and assists in establishing self-help programs. It maintains a library and is also an advocate for cancer patients. It publishes numerous newsletters and resource guides.

MAKE TODAY COUNT

101fi South Union Street
Alexandria, VA 22314
[no phone]

Through 200 local groups this organization helps people discuss the realities of life-threatening diseases. It sponsors a speakers bureau and offers referrals. Founded in 1974, it publishes the bimonthly *Make Today Count Newsletter*. There is a membership fee.

NATIONAL COALITION FOR CANCER SURVIVORSHIP

1010 Wayne Avenue 6th Floor
Silver Spring, MD 20910
301-650-8868

Founded in 1986, the coalition provides support and information to institutions and individuals. It sponsors data collection and a speakers bureau. Its publications include a newsletter. It also offers informational assistance on employment rights and insurance issues.

R.A. BLOCH CANCER FOUNDATION

H & R Bloch Building 4410 Main
Kansas City, MO 64111
816-932-8453

The foundation sponsors a Cancer Hot Line in selected cities to match patients for support and referrals. It publishes the quarterly *Cancer Hot Line News*.

SUSAN G. KOMEN BREAST CANCER FOUNDATION

5005 LBJ, Suite 370
Dallas, TX 75244
214-450-1777
800-462-9273

This organization was founded in 1982 and directs its education and research efforts at both patients and professionals. It also maintains a speakers bureau.

Y-ME NATIONAL ORGANIZATION FOR BREAST CANCER INFORMATION & SUPPORT

c/o Sharon Green
212 West Van Buren
Chicago, IL 60607-3908
312-986-8338
800-221-2141

Founded in 1978, this organization provides peer support and counseling, referrals, technical assistance, and a 24-hour hotline [312-986-8228]. Its publications include a newsletter.

CYSTIC FIBROSIS

CYSTIC FIBROSIS FOUNDATION

6931 Arlington Road, No. 200
Bethesda, MD 20814
301-951-4422
800-344-4823

The foundation provides research on the disease as well as the education and care of patients and their families. It sponsors 60 local groups.

DIABETES

AMERICAN DIABETES ASSOCIATION

National Center
1660 Duke Street
Alexandria, VA 22314
703-549-1500
800-232-3472

With over 800 local groups, the association promotes research and education, maintains a library, and assists in the exchange of information about the disease. Founded in 1940, it has a variety of publications, including the monthly *Diabetes Forecast*. There is a membership fee.

JUVENILE DIABETES FOUNDATION INTERNATIONAL

432 Park Avenue South
New York, NY 10016
212-785-9500
800-533-2873

This organization, founded in 1970, supports research and provides counseling, support, and education to diabetic children and their families. It publishes *Countdown*, a quarterly.

DISABILITY & INDEPENDENT LIVING

ACCENT ON INFORMATION

PO Box 700
Bloomington, IL 61702
309-378-2961

Founded in 1972, this organization provides computerized retrieval of information on problems, products, and services for the handicapped. Its sponsoring publication is the quarterly *Accent on Living*.

CLEARINGHOUSE ON DISABILITY INFORMATION

U.S. Department of Education
Office of Special Education &
Rehabilitation Services
Switzer Bldg., Room 3132

Washington, D.C. 20202-2524
202-205-8241
800-205-8241

The clearinghouse was founded in 1973 to respond to inquiries on Federally funded programs. It publishes the *Pocket Guide for Federal Help for People with Disabilities* and *Summary of Existing Legislation for People with Disabilities*.

DISABLED AMERICAN VETERANS

PO Box 14301
Cincinnati, OH 45250-0301
606-441-7300

This organization was founded in 1920 and now has over 2500 local groups. It provides service to disabled veterans and their families, including counseling and help with claims and benefits. It publishes the monthly *DAV Magazine*. There is a membership fee.

NATIONAL CENTER FOR DISABILITY SERVICES

201 I.U. Willets Road
Albertson, NY 11507
516-747-5400

Founded in 1952, the center has five units offering educational, vocational, social, and recreational opportunities for the disabled.

LEARNING HOW

PO Box 35481
Charlotte, NC 28235
704-376-4735

Founded in 1979, this organization acts as a referral service and employment agency for people with physical disabilities.

NATIONAL ASSOCIATION OF THE PHYSICALLY HANDICAPPED

Bethesda Scarlet Oaks, No. 117
440 Lafayette Avenue
Cincinnati, OH 45220-1000
513-961-8040

The association was founded in 1958 and promotes the overall welfare of handicapped persons. It publishes the quarterly *NAPH National Newsletter*. There is a membership fee.

NATIONAL CENTER FOR YOUTH WITH DISABILITIES

University of Minnesota
Adolescent Health Program
Box 721
420 Delaware Street Southeast
Minneapolis, MN 55455
612-626-2825
800-333-6293

The center was founded in 1986 to provide information and resources to adolescents and young adults with chronic illness or developmental disabilities. Focusing on adolescents, their families and educators, their aim is to assist in dealing with the transition from adolescence to adult life. Publications include a newsletter, *Connections*.

NATIONAL COUNCIL ON INDEPENDENT LIVING

2111 Wilson Boulevard
Suite 405
Arlington, VA 22201
703-525-3406

Aimed at both centers and individuals, the council provides support and technical assistance, education, and maintains a speakers bureau. Founded in

1982, its publications include the quarterly *NCIL Newsletter*. There is a membership fee.

NATIONAL EASTER SEAL SOCIETY

230 W. Monroe Suite 1800
Chicago, IL 60606-4802
312-726-6200
800-221-6827

Founded in 1919, the society operates numerous state and local centers to aid people with disabilities. They are involved in the full spectrum of advocacy and education. A catalog of both print and audio-visual materials is available by request.

NATIONAL INFORMA-TION CENTER FOR CHILDREN & YOUTH WITH DISABILITIES

PO Box 1492
Washington, D.C. 20013-1492
202-884-8200
800-695-0285

The center was founded in 1970 and provides information on the educational rights and special services available to children with disabilities. It also serves as a liaison with local organizations. Its publications include the annual *Disability Fact Sheet*.

NATIONAL ORGANIZA-TION ON DISABILITY

910 16th Street NW, Suite 600
Washington, D.C. 20006
202-293-5960

Founded in 1986, this organization provides public information and workshops on improved access for the disabled. Its publications include the quarterly *The Report*.

PARENTS HELPING PARENTS

3041 Olcott Street
Santa Clara, CA 95054
408-727-5775

This group was formed in 1976 to help families dealing with special needs children, including those with chronic illness. It maintains a library and speakers bureau and provides a variety of educational services. Its publications include a newsletter. There is a membership fee.

RESEARCH & TRAINING CENTER ON INDEPENDENT LIVING

University of Kansas
Room 4089 Dole
Lawrence, KS 66045
913-8644095

Founded in 1980, the center provides training and technical assistance and maintains a library. A catalog of publications and pamphlets is available by request.

EMPHYSEMA

See AMERICAN LUNG ASSOCIATION above.

HEARING LOSS

ALEXANDER GRAHAM BELL ASSOCIATION FOR THE DEAF

3417 Volta Place NW
Washington, D.C. 20007-2778
202-337-5220

Founded in 1890, this large organization provides total coverage for both hearing impaired patients and professionals through a network of both state and local groups. It publishes a wide variety of journals and newsletters. There is a membership fee.

AMERICAN ASSOCIATION FOR THE DEAF-BLIND

814 Thayer Avenue
Room 302
Silver Spring, MD 20910
301-588-6545 (TTY)
301-588-8705 (FAX)

The Association was founded in 1937 to encourage independent living for the deaf and blind. It has a library and provides referrals. It publishes *Deaf-Blind American* quarterly, in several formats. There is a membership fee.

HELEN KELLER NATIONAL CENTER FOR DEAF-BLIND YOUTHS & ADULTS

111 Middle Neck Road
Sands Point, NY 11050
516-944-8900
516-944-8637 (TTY)

With ten regional groups, the center provides evaluation, support, training, and rehabilitation, as well as a resource center. Founded in 1969, it publishes the annual *Directory of Agencies & Organizations Serving Deaf-Blind Individuals*.

NATIONAL ASSOCIATION OF THE DEAF

814 Thayer Avenue
Silver Spring, MD 20910
301-587-1788

Founded in 1880, and with 51 affiliated state associations, this organization serves as a clearinghouse, advocacy, and education group. Its publications include the *NAD Broadcaster*, the *Deaf American* and others. There is a membership fee.

HEART DISEASE STROKE

AMERICAN HEART ASSOCIATION STROKE CONNECTION

7272 Greenville Avenue
Dallas, TX 75231-4596
800-553-6321

This large network of local support groups has grown to over 1000 since its founding in 1979. It serves those recovering from a stroke as well as health care professionals. It also is a clearinghouse of information and trains caregivers through its Stroke Outreach Program. It publishes the bimonthly magazine *Stroke Connection*, and the aphasia newsletter *Stroke of Luck*.

THE MENDED HEARTS, INC.

7272 Greenville Avenue
Dallas, TX 75231
214-706-1442

Founded in 1951, there are over 250 local support groups for persons with heart disease, their families and friends. *Heartbeat* is published quarterly. There is a membership fee.

NATIONAL STROKE ASSOCIATION

8480 East Orchard Road
Suite 1000
Englewood, CO 80111-5015
303-771-1700

The Association, founded in 1984, has 5 state groups and provides guidance in developing local support groups. It also has a variety of educational programs and is developing an information

and referral hotline. It publishes *Be Stroke Smart* monthly.

STROKE CLUBS, INTERNATIONAL

805 12th Street
Galveston, TX 77550
409-762-1022

Founded in 1968 to provide mutual aid to stroke victims, this organization maintains a list of over 800 clubs in the United States. It publishes two annual bulletins.

ILEITIS/COLITIS

CROHN'S & COLITIS FOUNDATION OF AMERICA, INC.

386 Park Avenue South
17th Floor
New York, NY 10016-8804
212-685-3440
800-343-3637

Founded in 1965, the Foundation has 73 local groups, runs workshops, and sponsors a speakers bureau. It publishes both a quarterly magazine and a newsletter *IBD News*. There is a membership fee.

LUPUS

THE AMERICAN LUPUS SOCIETY

260 Maple Court Suite 123
Ventura, CA 93003
805-339-0443
800-331-1802

The Society was founded in 1973 to increase public awareness and knowledge of lupus. It assists patients and families through local chapters and support groups. It publishes the quarterly *Lupus Today* and a newsletter. There is a membership free.

THE L.E. SUPPORT CLUB
8039 Nova Ct.
North Charleston, SC 29420
803-764-1769

This organization, founded in 1984, offers emotional support and self-help education through a newsletter and correspondence. It publishes a newsletter, *LE Beacon*. There is a membership fee.

LUPUS FOUNDATION OF AMERICA
4 Research Place
Suite 180
Rockville, MD 20850-3226
301-670-9292
800-558-0121

By far the largest of the three lupus support organizations, the foundation was founded in 1977. It provides education, services and support for patients. It publishes a quarterly magazine, *Lupus News*, and a newsletter. There is a membership fee.

MULTIPLE SCLEROSIS

NATIONAL MULTIPLE SCLEROSIS SOCIETY
733 3rd Avenue
New York, NY 10017
212-986-3240
800-344-4867

The society has both local and regional groups. Founded in 1946, it supports a broad range of programs, including the quarterly magazine *Inside MS*. There is a membership fee.

MUSCULAR DYSTROPHY

MUSCULAR DYSTROPHY ASSOCIATION
3300 East Sunrise Drive
Tucson, AZ 85718
602-529-2000

Founded in 1950, the association has 154 local chapters and provides services through them. It publishes the quarterly newsletter, *Quest*.

PARKINSON'S DISEASE

PARKINSON'S DISEASE FOUNDATION
William Black Medical Research Building
Columbia-Presbyterian Medical Center
650 West 168th Street
New York, NY 10032
212-923-4700
800-457-6676

The foundation has 400 local groups which disseminate information and provide family counseling. In existence since 1957, it publishes the *PDF Newsletter*.

PARKINSON'S SUPPORT GROUPS OF AMERICA
11376 Cherry Hill Road
No. 204
Beltsville, MD 20705
301-937-1545

This group, founded in 1981, publishes *PSGA Update* newsletter, once or twice a year.

SCLERODERMA

SCLERODERMA FEDERATION
Peabody Office Building
One Newbury Street
Peabody, MA 01960
508-535-6600

The Federation, founded in 1973, is aimed at both patients and professionals. It provides support and education, as well as sponsoring research and a speakers bureau. It publishes a quarterly newsletter *The Beacon*. There is a membership fee.

SCLERODERMA INTERNATIONAL FOUNDATION
704 Garden Center Road
New Castle, PA 16101
412-652-3109

This organization provides a support network for patients, their family and friends, as well as professionals. It also supports research and education efforts. Founded in 1971, its publications include a newsletter.

SCLERODERMA RESEARCH FOUNDATION
Box 200
Columbus, NJ 08022
609-261-2200

Although primarily aimed at supporting medical research, the foundation is also developing a network of support centers. It was founded in 1978 and publishes a newsletter. There is a membership fee.

SCLERODERMA FEDERATION CALIFORNIA
8852 Enloe Avenue
Garden Grove, CA
92644
714-892-5297

Founded in 1989, this organization is expanding its network of informational and support groups from southern California to cover the entire state. Its publications include a newsletter. There is a membership fee.

UNITED SCLERODERMA FOUNDATION
PO Box 399
Watsonville, CA 95077-0399
408-728-2202
800-722-4673

With 65 regional groups providing education and support, the foundation has been in existence since 1975. It publishes a quarterly newsletter.

SIGHT LOSS

AMERICAN COUNCIL OF THE BLIND
1155 15th Street NW, Suite 720
Washington, D.C. 20005
202-467-5081
800-424-8666

Founded in 1961, the council is a membership group of blind and visually impaired people, as well as an information clearinghouse. It publishes *Braille Forum* on a monthly basis.

COUNCIL OF CITIZENS WITH LOW VISION
1400 North Drake Road, No. 218
Kalamazoo, MI 49006
616-381-9566
800-733-2258

The council has formed 10 state organizations since its founding in 1978. It provides support, education and self-help instruction to help people maximize the use of their low vision. It publishes the quarterly *CCLV Newsletter*. There is a membership fee.

PREVENT BLINDNESS AMERICA

500 East Remington Road
Schaumburg, IL 60173-5611
708-843-2020
800-331-2020

Founded in 1908, the society sponsors a wide range of programs including the National Center for Sight's *Infoline*.

SPINAL CORD INJURY & PARALYSIS

AMERICAN PARALYSIS ASSOCIATION

500 Morris Avenue
Springfield, NJ 07081
201-379-2690
800-225-0292 (General information)

Founded in 1979, the association encourages and supports research and operates a hotline providing information and support. Its publications include a newsletter. There is a membership fee.

NATIONAL SPINAL CORD INJURY ASSOCIATION

545 Concord Avenue, Suite 29
Cambridge, MA 02138
617-441-8500
800-962-9629

A large organization in existence since 1948, the association encourages research and education, and provides a network, referrals, counseling, and a library. Its publications include *A Resource Directory*. There is a membership fee.

PARALYZED VETERANS OF AMERICA

801 18th Street NW
Washington, D.C. 20006
202-872-1300

Founded in 1946, and now having 40 regional groups, this organization provides help, information, and advocacy for paralyzed veterans. It also sponsors a variety of wheelchair sporting events. Its publications include the monthly *Paraplegia News*. There is a membership fee.

SPINAL CORD SOCIETY

Wendell Road
Fergus Falls, MN 56537
218-739-5252

Over 170 local groups have been formed since the society's founding in 1978. The focus is on data collection and research towards finding a cure, rather than rehabilitation. It publishes the monthly *Spinal Cord Society Newsletter*. A subscription to the newsletter covers membership.

INDEX

OTHER ULYSSES PRESS
HEALTH BOOKS

COUNT OUT CHOLESTEROL
Art Ulene, M.D. and Val Ulene, M.D.

>   Complete with counter and detailed dietary plan,
>   this companion resource to the Count Out Cholesterol
>   Cookbook shows how to design a cholesterol-lowering
>   program that's right for you. $12.95

COUNT OUT CHOLESTEROL COOKBOOK
Art Ulene, M.D. and Val Ulene, M.D.

>   A companion guide to *Count Out Cholesterol*, this
>   book shows you how to bring your cholesterol levels
>   down with the help of 250 gourmet recipes. $14.95

HOW TO CUT YOUR MEDICAL BILLS
Art Ulene, M.D. and Val Ulene, M.D.

>   This handy book offers insiders tips known only to
>   health professionals and savvy patients. It shows
>   how to save money on doctor bills, hospital costs,
>   drug prescriptions, and much more. $11.95

THE VITAMIN STRATEGY
Art Ulene, M.D. and Val Ulene, M.D.

>   A game plan for good health, this book helps read-
>   ers design a vitamin and mineral program tailored
>   to their individual needs. $11.95

DISCOVERY PLAY
Art Ulene, M.D. and Steven Shelov, M.D.

>   This book guides parents through the first three
>   years of their child's life, offering play activity with
>   a special emphasis on nurturing self-esteem. $9.95

LOSE WEIGHT WITH DR. ART ULENE
Art Ulene, M.D.

> This best-selling weight-loss book offers a 28-day program for taking off the pounds and keeping them off forever. $12.95

LAST WISHES: A HANDBOOK TO GUIDE YOUR SURVIVORS
Lucinda Page Knox, M.S.W. and Michael D. Knox, Ph.D.

> A simple do-it-yourself workbook, *Last Wishes* helps people put their affairs in order and eases the burden on their survivors. It allows them to plan their own funeral and leave final instructions for survivors. $12.95

IRRITABLE BOWEL SYNDROME: A NATURAL APPROACH
Rosemary Nicol

> This book offers a natural approach to a problem millions of sufferers have. The author clearly defines the symptoms and offers a dietary and stress-reduction program for relieving the effects of this disease. $9.95

KNOW YOUR BODY: THE ATLAS OF ANATOMY
Introduction by Trevor Weston, M.D.

> Designed to provide a comprehensive and concise guide to the structure of the human body, *Know Your Body* offers more than 250 color illustrations. An easy-to-follow road map of the human body. $11.95

MOOD FOODS
William Vayda

> *Mood Foods* shows how the foods you eat can influence your emotions, behavior, and personality. It also explains how a proper diet can help to alleviate such common complaints as PMS, hyperactivity, mood swings, and stress. $9.95

PANIC ATTACKS: A NATURAL APPROACH
Shirley Trickett

> Addresses the problem of panic attacks using a
> holistic approach. With a simple program focusing
> on diet, breathing, and relaxation, the book helps
> you understand this phenomenon and teaches how
> to prevent future attacks. $8.95

BREAKING THE AGE BARRIER: STAYING YOUNG, HEALTHY AND VIBRANT
Helen Franks

> Drawing on the latest medical research, *Breaking
> the Age Barrier* explains how the proper lifestyle
> can stop the aging process and make you feel
> youthful and vital. $12.95

THE BOOK OF KOMBUCHA: UNLOCKING THE SECRETS OF THE 2000-YEAR-OLD CHINESE "TEA MUSHROOM"
Beth Ann Petro

> *The Book of Kombucha* explains the health benefits
> of the "tea mushroom" while answering the con-
> cerns surrounding this alternative health treatment.
> Draws on up-to-date research and explains how to
> grow and use Kombucha. $11.95

*To order these or other Ulysses Press books call 800-377-2542 or
write to Ulysses Press, P.O. Box 3440, Berkeley, CA 94703-
3440. All retail orders are shipped free of charge. California resi-
dents must include sales tax. Allow two to three weeks for
delivery.*

ABOUT THE AUTHOR

Dr. JoAnn LeMaistre is a member of the clinical faculty of the Stanford University School of Medicine who has lectured widely. She is a practicing clinical psychologist who specializes in working with patients who have chronic medical illness or disability. Her own path toward able-heartedness includes parenthood, work, and multiple sclerosis. She is a recipient of the Distinguished Humanitarian Award from the California Psychological Association and the Mother of the Year Award from her local multiple sclerosis society.